"Adrenal burnout isn't your fault in our fast-faster society, yet its ramifications can stall fat loss and create weight loss resistance. In *The Adrenal Reset Diet,* Dr. Alan Christianson provides practical, easy-to-implement strategies to reset your adrenals, lose fat fast, and restore optimal health."

—JJ Virgin, *New York Times* bestselling author
of *The Virgin Diet,* JJVirgin.com

"Dr. Alan Christianson finally proves that weight gain is not your fault. The key to getting lean is to reset your inner clock, not to struggle and starve. His diet gives you the definitive formula to lose weight and thrive."

—Sara Gottfried, MD, *New York Times* bestselling author
of *The Hormone Cure,* SaraGottfriedMD.com

"In *The Adrenal Reset Diet,* Dr. Alan Christianson sheds new light on weight loss by teaching you how you can use carbohydrate and protein cycling along with resistant starch to balance your hormone levels and decrease your blood sugar and insulin levels. A must-read for anyone who lives in our modern stressed-out world."

—Jayson and Mira Calton, authors of *Naked Calories*
and *Rich Food, Poor Food,* CaltonNutrition.com

"As Dr. Christianson so eloquently explains, simple change in your diet and lifestyle can make a profound difference in your weight, energy, and overall well-being. It's not just what you eat, but *when you eat it.* The recipes are delicious and easy to prepare, and the meals, never boring. His recommendations are easy to follow and implement, scientifically based, and they yield rapid rewards. You owe it to your health to read this!"

—Hyla Cass, MD, integrative physician, author of
8 Weeks to Vibrant Health, CassMD.com

"*The Adrenal Reset Diet* is a breakthrough book with real solutions to optimize adrenal function and increase your energy, lose weight, and feel balanced. Dr. Christianson has a wealth of knowledge, and we are fortunate to have this book that shares his experience and wisdom. He lays it out with an easy-to-follow and results-driven approach."

—Dr. Trevor Cates, creator of the 21-Day Healthy
Habits Challenge, DrTrevorCates.com

"Whether you're struggling with your weight, living a high-stress lifestyle, or just not feeling like yourself, you *must* read this book. Using the latest cutting-edge science, Dr. Christianson masterfully proves that obesity is not just a matter of poor diet, inactivity, or lack of "willpower," but a survival response instigated by your own body. Find out exactly how to press the reset button and transform your body from stressed and fat to thriving and fit. Highly recommended!"

—Sean Croxton, host of *Underground Wellness*, UndergroundWellness.com

"*The Adrenal Reset Diet* gives us a badly needed brand-new perspective on why people gain weight. These ideas are timely and will help thousands understand how to safely use carbs and manage their lives to heal their adrenals."

—Kevin Gianni, health author, activist, and blogger, RenegadeHealth.com

"The secret to health isn't found in a crash diet, ab-sculpting gizmo, magical fat loss pill. It's our lifestyle that is out of sync with the ancient intelligence of our biology, and we're suffering as a result. Dr. Alan's dietary hacks, adrenal tonics, breathing exercises, and relaxation techniques show you how you can retune your body to truly thrive. Do yourself a favor and read this book."

—Abel James, author of *The Wild Diet* and host of
Fat-Burning Man, FatBurningMan.com

"I am so excited that Dr. Christianson has used his years of clinical experience and research to write *The Adrenal Reset Diet*. I've seen immense benefit from working with Dr. Christianson to improve my own health and have tried many of the protocols he outlines in this book. *The Adrenal Reset Diet* provides hope and real solutions to those who struggle with yo-yo dieting, hormonal problems, and stress. This awesome resource is full of practical advice and tips without any hype. I will definitely be recommending this book to family, friends, and readers."

—Katie of WellnessMama.com

"The adrenal glands are central to so much of what's going on with our health today. The great news is that we can fix dysfunction of our adrenal glands with diet. The revolutionary part of Dr. Christianson's new book is using a diet to repair the adrenals to help with weight loss. He has proven his method with a scientific study of his patients, which makes his new diet that much more likely to work for you!"

—Jennifer Landa, MD, author of *The Sex Drive Solution for Women*, creator of the Three Weeks to Endless Energy program, DrJenniferLanda.com

"A must-read if you suffer from weight gain, exhaustion, or stress. Dr. Alan Christianson has outlined a simple yet highly effective diet to restore balance, health, and sanity!"

—Cynthia Pasquella, CCN, bestselling author of *PINK Method* and *The Hungry Hottie Cookbook*, founder of the Institute of Transformational Nutrition, CynthiaPasquella.com

"Everyone is doing too much and ultimately they pay the physical price. Dr. Alan Christianson has formulated an easy-to-follow dietary solution to help reset the overworked adrenals and create lasting fat loss. *Thumbs up!* for this great approach!"

—Marcelle Pick, OB/GYN, NP, owner of Women to Women, author of *The Core Balance Diet* and *Is It Me or My Adrenals?*, MarcellePick.com

"If you've ever unsuccessfully tried to lose weight, or you've tried diets that haven't worked, or you've been confused by experts offering conflicting advice, or you simply don't think any new weight loss solution will work for you . . . then you *must* read this book. In *The Adrenal Reset Diet,* Dr. Alan Christianson explains how our adrenal glands control a switch that causes us to burn fat and feel energized . . . *or* . . . store fat and feel tired. The secret to weight loss is in our adrenal glands. After decades of research and over 75,000 patient-care visits, Dr. Alan shows you that no matter how long you've struggled with your weight, and no matter how many diets have failed you, it has *not* been your fault. It's simply the fact that your body has been under stress from a list of factors described in this book. The good news is Dr. Alan takes you by the hand and shows you how to put your adrenal glands into the "fat-burning" mode so you lose weight and feel energized. If you want to start losing weight today and feeling great, read this book now."

—Joe Polish, founder of the Genius Network, JoePolish.com

"*The Adrenal Reset Diet* eloquently shows us that being overweight is not simply a matter of eating less and moving more. Nor is it due to zero willpower! As a nutritionist who works with anxious women, many of whom are stress eaters with burned-out adrenals, I know this book will be a valuable resource for me and my clients."

—Trudy Scott, CN, author of *The Antianxiety Food Solution*, AntianxietyFoodSolution.com

"Dr. Christianson's newest book, *The Adrenal Reset Diet*, is revolutionary (yet scientific) and teaches the reader how to simply lose weight, feel better, and finally get your hormones balanced. Easy to read and understand, this book is a must-read!"

—Leanne Ely, CNC, *New York Times* bestselling author, SavingDinner.com

"If you feel tired all the time, can't seem to lose those extra pounds around the waist, have trouble sleeping, and are overwhelmed with stress, Dr. Alan Christianson's new book, *The Adrenal Reset Diet*, will explain in detail the root cause of your symptoms AND provide very simple but profound strategies to restore your energy and vitality! This is a must-read on how to thrive in the modern world!"

—Dr. Susanne Bennett, author of *The 7-Day Allergy Makeover*, host of *The Wellness for Life* radio show, and creator of the Heal Your Gut, Heal Your Life program, DrSusanne.com

"In *The Adrenal Reset Diet*, Dr. Alan Christianson clarifies the true cause of the obesity epidemic and provides a brilliant plan to shift from stressed and overweight to trim and thriving. If you are stressed and can't lose weight, you must read this book."

—Steven Masley, MD, FAHA, FACN, FAAFP, CNS, bestselling author of *The 30-Day Heart Tune-Up*, HeartTuneUp.com

**strategically cycle
carbs and proteins
to lose weight,
balance hormones,
and move from
stressed to thriving**

the

adrenal
reset
diet

ALAN CHRISTIANSON, NMD

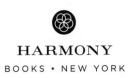

HARMONY

BOOKS · NEW YORK

The material in this book is for informational purposes only and not intended as a substitute for the advice and care of your physician. As with all new weight loss or weight maintenance regimens, the nutrition and wellness program described in this book should be followed only after first consulting with your physician to make sure it is appropriate for your individual circumstances. Keep in mind that nutritional needs vary from person to person, depending on age, sex, health status, and total diet. The author and the publisher expressly disclaim responsibility for any adverse effects that may result from the use or application of the information contained in this book.

Published in the United States by Harmony Books, an imprint of the Crown Publishing Group, a division of Random House LLC, a Penguin Random House Company, New York. www.crownpublishing.com

Harmony Books is a registered trademark, and the Circle colophon is a trademark of Random House LLC.

Library of Congress Cataloging-in-Publication Data
Christianson, Alan.
The adrenal reset diet: strategically cycle carbs and proteins to lose weight, balance hormones, and move from stressed to thriving / Alan Christianson, NMD; foreword by Sara Gottfried, MD.
1. Weight loss.   2. Weight loss—Endocrine aspects.   3. Metabolism—Regulation.   4. Adrenal glands.   5. Reducing diets.   I. Title.
RM222.2.C4839 2014
613.2'82—dc23   2014022662

ISBN 978-0-8041-4053-9
eBook ISBN 978-0-8041-4054-6

Printed in the United States of America

Book design by Ralph Fowler
Jacket design by Jess Morphew
Illustration on page 30 by Celestina Christianson

10 9 8 7 6 5 4 3 2 1

First Edition

contents

foreword

Science tells us that losing weight is 80 percent diet and 20 percent exercise, but after twenty years of medical practice, I don't buy it. My friend and colleague Dr. Alan Christianson has an explanation that makes far more sense: the reason you're having trouble losing weight is that your hormonal rhythms are out of whack, specifically stress hormones such as cortisol. This fact leads skillfully to the fix: reset your adrenal rhythms, stress hormones, and cortisol pattern.

Dr. C's book takes you by the hand and shows you how to fix the problem and get lean. But first you may wonder (like David Byrne): How did I get here? Alan expertly describes how getting fat is a survival response from our DNA. When you're running around, crazed by stress, you turn on the fat storage genes and create havoc with your stress hormones. When the survival response disrupts the adrenal rhythms, you gain weight. As if that weren't bad enough, restricting food and over-exercising doesn't help because they deepen the survival response; your body fears you're in for a famine so it shuts down your metabolism.

I know this pattern very well after living through it myself as a working mom. Have you heard the analogy that life is like a four-burner stove? It goes like this: One burner represents family, another is friends, another is health, and the last one is work. You can't have all four burners going at once. To manage life skillfully, you need to have three out of four burners in the "on" position. If you want to be very successful, you have to choose two of the four burners.

Sure enough, when I was in my thirties, I tried to keep all four burners going, and flipped my body into survival mode. I got fat, frazzled, and frumpy. Maybe you find yourself in a similar situation.

It took applying my world-class medical education to my own misery to sort out my disrupted biology. I was fortunate to write a book about it, a bestseller called *The Hormone Cure*. I discovered, through my own healing, and after losing twenty-five pounds, that the root cause of my fatness was my stress-crazed life and broken adrenal rhythms. It made me store belly fat as if I were an Irish farmer in the midst of a famine and didn't know when my next meal would be; it robbed me of the happy brain chemicals like serotonin; and it aged me (and my DNA) prematurely.

truth can be frustrating yet effective

Truth is sacred and liberating, but initially, it can be frustrating—especially when it involves changing the way you eat and move. That's where Dr. Alan Christianson excels. He's like a knight in shining armor with a white doctor's coat. Alan offers his patients, and now you, the bold yet effective truth about how to craft a plate and a life scientifically designed to heal your broken metabolism.

Dr. C also models his powerful message every minute of his life.

paging dr. alan christianson

I met Alan many years ago at a health conference hosted by a mutual friend, JJ Virgin. At the time, Dr. C was a highly regarded Arizona-based Naturopathic Medical Doctor (NMD) who specialized in natural endocrinology with a focus on thyroid and adrenal disorders.

I liked Dr. C so much that I went to visit him the next time I gave a speech in Scottsdale. In his typical fashion, Alan brought me from the airport to his clinic, Integrative Healthcare, and gave me intravenous glutathione. My adrenals perked right up. That night, after my dinnertime speech, I stayed with Alan and his lovely family in Scottsdale. He served me the food he describes in this new book and didn't serve me the bad stuff, such as coffee or wine. After eight hours of sleep, I woke up to the fragrant smell of Dr. C cooking a low-carb breakfast of pastured eggs, sausage, and organic greens while his wife performed beauty pageant leg lifts, preparing for a bathing suit photo shoot. By the time I hit the kitchen with my mouth watering, he had a two-hour hike planned for us, and had packed filtered water, trekking poles, and a nutrient-dense lunch. I eyed him a little skeptically as he described the various hiking options: we could hike for four hours and go straight to the airport afterward, or take a more leisurely two-hour hike and have time for lunch. I chose the latter. Alan took me on a favorite hike in the McDowell Mountains.

I mention the visit because it demonstrates Dr. C's searing wisdom and how he walks the talk. Alan puts it all together in a way that's incredibly valuable for people who seek to lose weight and feel better fast.

Kindly allow me to unpack the various pieces of the puzzle that he believes contribute to our adrenal health—and natural weight maintenance:

- Intravenous glutathione is one of the best antioxidants—it removes the rust of modern life.

- The lack of alcohol (Alan doesn't drink on a regular basis, and alcohol uses up your internal store of glutathione).

- A low-carb breakfast supports your innate cortisol curve.

- The long hike was designed to improve my glycogen sensitivity, which is one of the body's ways of balancing glucose. You see, my tendency is to make too much cortisol in the morning (above the ideal level), and Alan explained that when I do long slow distance (LSD) exercise, I will improve my adrenal rhythm in the morning. Even cooler is the fact that I only need to do LSD such as hiking or biking a few times per month, for three-plus hours.

- Trekking poles reduce pressure from hiking. Not only do they provide better balance and footing, they also decrease the amount of stress on your legs and joints on downhill slopes. When climbing uphill, trekking poles transfer some of your weight to your shoulders, arms, and back, which can lower leg fatigue and add thrust to your climbs. Overall, trekking poles can reduce compressive force on the knees by up to 25 percent.

Fortunately, you don't need to travel to Phoenix to get Alan's nurturing guidance—you hold in your hands his keys to the kingdom.

how dr. alan christianson can help you

I've found that about 90 percent of the people in my functional medicine practice have a problem with cortisol. This is a major issue—as Dr. C says, a bad cortisol slope is more dangerous than smoking, documented in the Whitehall II study from 2011.

What role does cortisol plays in metabolism? Cortisol is a catabolic chemical, meaning it causes wear and tear if it is too high, which in turn can make you gain weight and crave sugar. Your adrenal glands do a delicate dance to maintain your weight, and when your cortisol is too high, the rhythm is disrupted.

How can you fix it? Alan has found a unique way to turn the ship around. If your problem is a flat cortisol plane—when your exhausted adrenals don't know how to maintain their normal cycle of high in the morning, low at night—eat a low-carb breakfast to aim for the ideal zone. Eat slow carbs at dinner (slow-to-digest yams are my favorites) to shut off cortisol so you can get the sleep you need to build and repair all that wear and tear from the day.

start with breakfast

I like eating a good, solid, protein-rich breakfast because I need my energy all day. I simply feel better. Alan's book made me realize just how strong an affect breakfast can have on my cortisol pattern. Nor should I borrow from tomorrow's energy today by drinking coffee all day just to get through. Every day should be like a profit center that is self-sustaining.

If you think you're doing yourself a favor by waking up to wholegrain cereal with low-fat milk and a cup of orange juice, you might want to think again. I know you were told at some point that it's a good breakfast, but the truth is that this standard breakfast is largely converted into triglycerides, contributing to a problem with cortisol. Before long you'll find yourself, as I did, with burned-out adrenal glands.

why old school no longer applies

We know that the old model of calorie counting and input versus output is failing for a lot of people, for a variety of reasons. Let's tease some of the stuff out. Even without being diabetic, you may develop insulin sensitivity and insulin resistance (your cells can't respond properly to insulin, so your body tries pumping out more), and as a result, you suffer from uncontrolled blood sugar. Then the dance continues: the adrenals jump in, trying to balance the blood sugar, and your cortisol goes out of control. Cortisol then tells your body, whoa, you're in trouble; store some fat for a rainy day. You know the end of this story: you gain weight.

This book is for you even if you're at a healthy weight, but you've got too much fat. We call that skinny-fat. You may look good in a T-shirt, but your belly is doughy. Not to scare you, but skinny-fat people have double the mortality rates of obese or overweight people.

Mainstream medicine doesn't believe in adrenal dysregulation. Many doctors will likely dismiss you if you try to discuss it with them. They'll say that your adrenal glands are either perfectly fine or in failure—there's no middle ground. In actuality, thousands of studies show that your adrenals and their functions in that in-between state can be associated with problems including obesity, high blood sugar, and insulin resistance.

dr. alan studied his protocol

Dr. C put his theories to the test and offered his program to a group of forty-two people last year: 88 percent female, with a mean age of forty-five. After thirty days, he found the following results with just his diet alone:

- weight loss of 9 pounds

- 2 percent drop in body fat

- 2 inches lost off the waist

- significant improvement in adrenal rhythm, as measured in 4-point or diurnal cortisol level

Remember, the most important thing is to have a good cortisol slope. If you have that, awesome. If your morning cortisol ramps up too high, then it is a matter of improving your glycogen sensitivity (how you store glucose). Sometimes you can spike morning cortisol above the ideal when your adrenals work harder for gluconeogenesis—the process of turning glucose from substances other than carbs into glucose. Here's where Alan's diet prescriptions come in. Exercise helps, too. While it's not as time efficient as burst training, LSD (long slow distance) training helps—do something that is ongoing for a few hours such as hiking or biking even a few times a month.

As I said earlier, I was my own worst enemy, going on all four burners—but then I applied my medical training to my broken body. Alan grew up as a fat kid. When he got tired of being different, he used his formidable intellect to overcome his challenge by reading dozens of nutrition and fitness books, then giving up sugar and beginning an exercise regimen. As an adult, he studied medicine, but realized that the mainstream medical approach doesn't have all the answers. As a naturopathic physician, Alan has transformed his lifelong love of learning and his education and experience into a surefire program to teach others how to use foods and nutrients for optimal health, including weight loss. Read it, get lean, and be well.

Sara Gottfried, MD
Berkeley, California

Sara Gottfried, MD, is one of the foremost authorities on how to reset hormones with evidence-based integration of modern medicine and ancient traditions. She is the author of *The Hormone Cure: Reclaim Balance, Sleep, Sex Drive, and Metabolism Naturally with The Gottfried Protocol.*

introduction

For years, you have been trying to improve your health. Despite your best efforts, your body does not cooperate. You have tried so many diet and exercise regimens, yet none has helped. Experts offer advice, but it is often contradictory. Some say you need to eat less sugar. Others say that the problem is you spend too much time indoors being sedentary. Many blame the illness on an indulgent personality.

By the way, the year is 1879 and you are suffering from tuberculosis.

As if the physical suffering from this illness were not enough, you have also suffered from guilt, thinking it was your fault. You were told you would get better if only you tried harder and stopped being lazy. You were told to think "better" thoughts, avoid certain foods, and do specific exercises. When you did not recover, instead of doubting the advice being handed out by the medical community, you found it easier to believe that you hadn't tried hard enough.

Many years before tuberculosis was widely understood, scientists like Benjamin Marten believed that it was caused, not by character, but by "wonderfully (tiny) living creatures."[1] Along with tuberculosis, other diseases were attributed to and blamed on personal character, including leprosy, smallpox, and cancer. Today we are in the same situation. Scientific information is out of sync with common beliefs. Even though science tells us that obesity is no more caused by character than tuberculosis was, many still continue to blame the victim. Not only is this hurtful but it also shifts the focus away from effective change.

Most people still believe that body weight is simply a matter of calories in via diet versus calories out via exercise. The assumption is that those who cannot lose weight are simply not trying hard enough. They are eating too much. They are slothful. It's their fault. Many popular slogans, magazine headlines, and book titles reflect this—"Eat Less, Move More"—or display a "Eat this, not that" mentality.

Yet this thinking is not up to date or correct for a large portion of the population. The correct information, however, is exciting: current research shows that what our bodies do with food depends on whether we are in a mode of thriving or surviving. A little set of glands, called the adrenals, is the master controller of these modes. Our adrenal glands control a switch that causes us to thrive, meaning we burn fat and feel energized, or just survive, meaning we store fat and feel tired. Processed food, pollutants, and the pressures of life can all push us into this survival mode. As important as survival mode is for short-term crises, if we spend too much time in it we gain weight, age faster, and die earlier.

I have a vivid memory of the moment when I got stuck in survival mode. I was in second grade and I believed that chocolate chip cookies were among the only things that made the world a better place. My family had just moved to work at a resort in northern Minnesota. One day, I managed to sneak a full handful of freshly baked chocolate chip cookies out of the kitchen. I vividly remember that somewhere past the third cookie, the pain of the recent move seemed to melt away. Over the next five years, I continued to gain weight, until one memorable day in seventh-grade gym class. A group of boys were debating who had the biggest boobs in our class. One of them managed to think outside the gender box and nominate me for the title. I already knew he was right, but I had hoped until then that others hadn't noticed.

After that painful day, I absolutely *had* to change. I read every book my library had that sounded promising. Most were on diet and exercise, but some were on health and medicine. After trying many different methods, I started to learn some things. One thing I learned was that if I starved myself or over-exercised, I only got hungrier. Sugar and bread were not too hard to give up—but only as long as I gave them up completely. My parents ordered me protein powders from a mail-order supplement company, and I used them for breakfast. Breathing exercises I learned from yoga seemed to make these changes easier to stick with.

Over the next year, the weight came off. Not only was I able to play sports but I also became one of the better athletes in our school. I was able to enjoy how great it felt to live fully and experience good health; several years later, a house fire taught me how easy it could be to lose that good feeling.

My family was fine, but we lost our pets and all of our possessions. To help us get back on our feet, I spent every moment I was not in school working at a restaurant. My stress levels were high, I had constant access to unhealthy food, and my exercise regime stopped. Soon, I was 30 pounds above target and completely out of shape.

Teenage angst led my next attempts at dieting, this time to become too extreme. I ate fewer foods and a lot less of them. Imagine living on a few servings of raw vegetables while being in school, working, and running 6 to 10 miles outdoors in the northern Minnesota winter.

I lost weight, but I soon found myself both unhealthy and depressed. Books came to my rescue again. One of the most memorable was the first edition of the *Textbook of Natural Medicine* by Michael Murray, ND. (Little did I know then that many years later Dr. Murray would become a personal friend and ask me to help author portions of the ninth edition of that same book.)

Dr. Murray's book taught me that I needed a more balanced diet, with more calories, adequate protein, healthy fats, and more mineral-rich foods. As a result, not only did my health flourish, but I also reconnected with my earlier interest in medicine. My life's focus shifted away from my personal needs; I wanted to deepen my understanding of nutrition and use it to help others the same way it had helped me. Finding a medical school whose curriculum focused on nutrition was a dream come true. My interest in the interplay of hormones and obesity emerged while I was working with a memorable young woman during my internship.

Jamie was a 16-year-old girl who was about to be forced to withdraw from high school. Jamie was bright and an eager student, but she was too sore and tired to get out of bed. After a really bad case of the flu the year before, nothing had been as before. Her weight shot up and all of her muscles hurt. At the time, most doctors did not recognize fibromyalgia as a real condition, but one doctor who did said that this was the culprit. Unfortunately, there was no known cure.

I realized that as much as my health had bothered me in the past, Jamie's condition was much worse. My supervising doctor let me spend time with Jamie's chart in the medical research library. I managed to piece together a few things: Jamie's symptoms were similar to those of thyroid disease; her mother and grandmother both had thyroid disease. The other doctors said this could not be the cause of Jamie's symptoms because her thyroid blood tests were normal. Yet I found studies showing that sometimes the common tests for thyroid function failed to show the disease when it was just starting.

My supervising doctors were willing to do more detailed tests, and these confirmed that Jamie was suffering from thyroid disease. Treating this condition allowed Jamie to get back to her studies and attend her prom. Although the thyroid treatment helped spur her initial weight loss, it took more investigation to get her back to her goal weight. I discovered that her thyroid disease had hurt her adrenal glands; I had suspected this because she was often dizzy from low blood pressure and she had strong salt cravings, and these were both signs of poor adrenal function. Once we identified this problem and helped coax her levels back to their optimal range, she was able to truly thrive again. After seeing Jamie get her life back, I became even more convinced that many puzzling conditions have a hormonal root cause.

Jamie has since grown up, gotten a degree, and is raising a beautiful family. To me, nothing is more important than being able to help someone like Jamie move to a place of better health and more happiness.

The program that is in your hands, *The Adrenal Reset Diet,* is the culmination of a child's frustration, decades of research, and over 75,000 patient-care visits.

The Adrenal Reset Diet really is different because it is not a "low-anything" diet—in fact, too little food and too much exercise can actually cause weight gain. Food is the cure, not the enemy. Some unique aspects that make my system work and that benefit you beyond weight loss, include:

- *Carbs are not forbidden;* instead, carbohydrates are cycled so you can reverse the effects of processed foods on visceral fat stores.

- *Circadian rhythms are fixed;* this helps you sleep better and allows your liver to help control your weight.

- *Clarity is restored through 5-minute rituals;* these keep the pressures of life (stress) from damaging your brain and raising your appetite.

Now we come to the most important part of this story, *you.* No matter how long you have struggled with your weight, or how many diets have failed you, *it has not been your fault.*

You have never lacked willpower or courage. You are not weak or indulgent. Your body has been under stress from processed food, pollution, and the pressures of life. It has been trying to help you survive the only way it knows how. Soon you will learn why this happens and how you can gently switch from surviving to *thriving.*

We all have something to share with the world, yet this is hard to realize when our health feels out of control. I know how amazing it is to be able to put a long struggle to the side and get on with your life, to realize its purpose and mission. How would your life be if nothing was holding you back? Let's find out.

Alan Christianson, NMD
Scottsdale, Arizona

why are we gaining weight?

ONE OF MY FAVORITE POSSESSIONS IS A COPY OF *TIME* MAGAzine from July 1969. The cover story is about the historic *Apollo 11* moon launch. The main picture in the story shows hundreds of people standing in an observation field, looking to the sky as the rocket lifts off. Recently, I looked again at the photo with a vague sense that there was something odd about it. After looking several times, I suddenly realized what it was: everyone in the crowd was unusually thin. The observers were mostly men, and they looked to be mostly in their early 40s.

In the 1960s, the average American male between the ages of 40 and 45 weighed 169 pounds. By the year 2000, that average weight was 196 pounds, nearly 30 pounds heavier.[1] A similar crowd today would look quite different yet again.

a global obesity crisis—the stats

By 2010, rates of obesity had increased yet more; over 69 percent of American adults had become overweight or obese. And the same changes had happened worldwide; the number of overweight and obese adults around the world began creeping up in the 1970s, and then it doubled between 1980 and 2008. *It is estimated that there are now over 1.4 billion adults in the world who are overweight.* For the first time in human history, deaths from obesity-related illnesses have surpassed deaths from all other causes, including malnutrition and infectious disease.

If these deaths were not bad enough, the costs of managing future decades of chronic diseases are projected to cripple the global economy. It is estimated that in the next twenty years, obesity-related diseases will cost the global economy in excess of $30 trillion. To put this into perspective, the 9/11 attacks on the United States, combined with the wars in Iraq and Afghanistan, are estimated to have cost roughly $5 trillion.[2]

There is no doubt that people are gaining weight faster than ever before, but why is this happening? Cutting-edge medical research has some good answers, but unfortunately most of the public and the majority of policymakers base their beliefs about obesity on theories we now know are not true. The popular view blames obesity on too many calories, too little willpower, and bad genes. *It's not that simple.*

the calorie theory: no longer in

Let's start with the calorie model for weight gain. It certainly is appealing in its simplicity: people gain weight because they eat more calories than they burn. Although the calorie model does reflect what happens to healthy people in controlled settings, it does not explain what happens when bodies are stressed and move into survival mode. During most of our past, stress came from immediate danger, such as predators trying to eat us or us having too little of our own food. Our genes adapted to stress by causing us to store food as fat rather than to burn it as fuel.

Even if it were true that heavier people just ate more than others do, this does not explain why, in the last few decades, people are suddenly seeming to eat more than ever. At best, the calorie model describes the situation; it does not explain the root cause. It's just like saying "People in the Third World earn less" describes the situation, but does not explain world poverty.

babies do not need willpower

Traci Mann, UCLA associate professor of psychology, evaluated thirty-one long-term studies to see how effective calorie-based weight-loss programs were over the long haul. She reported that even for the minority of people who did lose weight, four years later, *83 percent of them were heavier than before they had started the program.* In fact, more than half of them gained 11 pounds or more *over* the weight they had lost.[3] If the problem was simply one of discipline, why did those who had enough discipline to lose weight then regain so much weight?

When presented with failures in dieting, many if not most people assume that those who did not succeed simply lacked willpower and did not try hard enough. They have no problem assuming that an adult's weight is a result of his or her conscious choices, yet few would hold this same idea if it were applied to infants or animals. When a baby cries for a bottle, is she acting out of hunger or because she is being indulgent? How about wild animals—does willpower govern their body weight? Yet the rate of obesity, and morbid obesity, in infants has multiplied several times over the last decade, and it continues to increase rapidly. For the first time ever, 6-month-old babies are becoming morbidly obese. This is happening despite there being no related changes to the types or amounts of food they are given.[4]

And this widespread obesity issue isn't affecting just the human population. In 2010, David Allison and colleagues evaluated weight changes spanning the last several decades in 20,000 animals from eight different species, including macaques, chimpanzees, vervets, marmosets, lab rats and mice, feral rats, and domestic dogs and cats. Some of the animals gaining weight lived in the wild, some were pets, and some were even on carefully measured diets. Shockingly, mid-life obesity had increased in *100 percent* of the species studied. One of our closest living relatives saw especially shocking changes. Despite living in zoos and having their diets and activity levels controlled, the weight of male and female chimpanzees had gone up by 33.2 and 37.2 percent per decade, respectively.[5] After evidence like this, the claim that obesity is a disease of willpower is completely unsupportable.

genes vs. jeans

Another popular belief about obesity is that it is caused by faulty genes. Many scientists say that the human body has had little major change in 200,000 years. Historically, we've seen populations suffer from weight loss due to malnutrition and famine, but global weight gain across many species has never happened before. Even if in the distant past there had been individual cases of weight gain, it was often limited to royalty. So how valid could be this idea about the role of genes in weight gain?

Genes *can* influence why one person may gain more weight than another, but familial genes alone cannot explain why weight gain has occurred all around the globe and to so many different living things. But *epigenetics,* a science that shows how our environment and genes interact, may hold some answers. Research in this area suggests that genes themselves may not be the culprits; instead, there may be ways the modern world has been changing our genes that is behind this global problem. What's most exciting is that there are steps in *The Adrenal Reset Diet* that can fight these negative modern influences and help you change your genes back.

surprising causes of weight gain

If the global weight explosion is not caused by too many calories, lack of personal responsibility, or bad genes, then what *is* the cause? To answer that question we need to think about what else has changed during this same time period. Many researchers have wrestled with these questions, and some common answers have emerged. To begin, within the last few decades our world has gotten more toxic, a lot noisier, and much faster paced. Our food has more sugar, less fiber, and many more chemicals. We spend less time in sunlight and we sleep less. We take more medications, feel less certain of our financial futures, and have fewer friends.

Although experts debate which of these culprits is the most important, they strongly agree that global weight gain is brought about by some combination of these changes. Because any one of these causes has such strong evidence linking it to obesity, researchers have become individually fixated on one cause or another.

When I dug into this problem, in my work as a doctor, I realized that the answer to the obesity epidemic would have to encompass all of the possible triggers. (To simplify, these triggers can be thought of as processed foods, pollutants, and the pressures of life.) There had to be *one* thing they all had in common. I also realized that, even though there may not be a single cause, there still could be a single way by which different causes trigger weight gain.

a unifying theory of obesity

What was the single thread running through all these factors? It started to become clear one day when I was studying how obesity is tied to adrenal hormones. It turns out that adrenal hormones control a switch that sends calories to your belly fat or to your muscles. In layperson's terms, when the switch is set to "fat," calories go to your fat cells, making them larger. This is not good. When the switch is set to "energy," calories go to your muscles, where they make energy. This is good. But why would our adrenal glands signal to our bodies to make our bellies fat?

They do it to protect us. When we are in danger, our muscles need to be able to burn large amounts of energy quickly, so we can run away or fight. Our muscles are unable to burn energy when they are storing energy, so your calories are sent away from them. Since these calories have to go somewhere, and since in our past "danger" often meant food shortages, our visceral fat (what we call belly fat, but is actually fat deposition around our organs) takes in these calories and stores them. This is survival mode, and it causes weight gain because our calories are taken from our muscles and placed in our fat cells.

In survival mode, most of us prefer foods that are higher in sugar, salt, and fat. In addition to causing us to gain weight regardless of what we eat, survival mode can cause us to want to eat more and to prefer foods that cause weight gain to happen even faster.

You can imagine that there is a switch in your body like the switch you use to turn on your lights. I think of it as the "fat switch"; and in survival mode, it is turned on. *The Adrenal Reset Diet* teaches you how to use everyday foods to reset your adrenal glands and turn that fat switch off for good. But to learn how to do this, it is important you have a better understanding of the survival mode.

survival mode is more than "stress"

Though we've come to think of stress as something we feel when we're under emotional pressure—a response to feeling too busy, overwhelmed with duties and the rush of modern life—the earliest definition of the word *stress* included anything that would trigger survival mode in an animal. This trigger, thus, includes physical and environmental stress, dietary stress, and mental stress. To understand how many different factors can add up and push our bodies to create fat, therefore, it is important to think of stress in this broader way.

All animals can maintain their body weights within a certain range, even when food intake goes up or down. This is regulated primarily by our adrenal glands. In response to stress, the adrenal glands release *cortisol* into the bloodstream. Whether we are surviving or thriving determines how the cortisol will act in our brain, liver, and belly fat. In survival mode, the cortisol causes us to slow down and store fat. When we are thriving, we eat for hunger and our bodies are able to adjust the metabolism to keep our weight healthy, even with minor amounts of stress. But when we get pushed into survival mode, this all changes and we become more apt to gain weight. Stress does not create weight gain until there is a disruption in this adrenal rhythm.

Why would being in survival mode lead to weight gain? The

lesson our genes learned during the last 200,000 years was that bad things do not happen during times of plenty. Stress usually meant danger, famine, or both. Our ancestors who stored fat during times of crisis survived better than those who did not. This means they were able to live and have babies, and share their gene pool with their descendants, us.

When we are under a constant state of adrenal stress, our bodies prepare for famine by burning fewer calories and storing fat around our organs—that *visceral fat* that was mention a little earlier in this chapter. Think of visceral fat as cash under the mattress. It is the quickest, most accessible fuel resource your body can have for a crisis. The fat on the hips, thighs, and under the skin is *subcutaneous fat*. It's more like savings bonds: a safe source of fuel, but we can't get to it very easily.

When a person is in survival mode, he or she will gain more visceral fat than an unstressed person eating the same number of calories. However, stress does not cause us to store more of the harmless subcutaneous fat below our skin, just the dangerous visceral fat around our organs. This is because our bodies rely on visceral fat as fuel during times of crisis. Not only that, the extra stress hormones prevent the body's organs from effectively using energy in the muscles or brain, leading to fatigue and depression.[6]

What about those people who lose their appetite when stressed?

TABLE 1.1. PROBLEMS THAT LEAD TO WEIGHT GAIN

PROBLEMS	PROCESSED FOOD	POLLUTANTS	PRESSURES OF LIFE
Details	Fructose Toxic proteins	Environmental Light	Relationships Work Finances
Consequences	Adrenal Fat Switch gets set to survival mode. Hunger increases, energy decreases, and food is stored as fat.		

It is true that not everyone gains pounds when under major stress, but those who do not gain scale weight still typically experience a loss of muscle mass and an increase in body fat.

If being in survival mode leads to weight gain, what triggers this reaction and what can you do about it? The known triggers come in three main categories: dietary, mental, and physical. Table 1.1 shows the three factors that lead to weight gain.

⮞ trigger #1: processed food

Processed foods in the modern diet can increase inflammation and disrupt blood sugar levels. This inflammation causes the body to make more cortisol to reduce that inflammation and control the blood sugar level in the same way as when the body makes more cortisol when it senses fright.

The main culprits of inflammation include fructose and toxic proteins. *Fructose* is a type of sugar that directly turns our fat switch to storage mode. It does this by activating liver enzymes with exotic names like c-JNK and 11-HSD, which make us store fat. *Toxic proteins* are proteins in our foods that are hard to break down all the way in normal digestion, and their unbroken parts are then attacked by the body's immune system. These proteins are found in dairy foods, eggs, and wheat, and they often can trigger inflammation. You know how you feel when you have the flu? That sick feeling is not from the virus but, rather, the inflammation caused by your immune system attacking that virus. That same inflammation is created when your immune system attacks the undigested parts of protein.

fructose

The modern diet differs in many ways from diets of the past. Of all the differences, the most significant may be the rate at which modern foods are absorbed. After chewing in the mouth and swallowing, food moves to our stomach, where acids digest it into smaller

evolution of the human diet

TIME FRAME	DIETARY STAPLES
200,000–10,000 BCE	Wild game, fresh vegetables, fresh fruits
10,000 BCE–1960 AD	Farm-raised animals and dairy, unprocessed grains, fresh vegetables, fresh fruits
1960–1980	Factory-raised animals and dairy, processed grains, canned vegetables, fruit juice
1980 to present	Factory-raised animals and dairy, high fructose corn syrup, processed grains

parts. This can be thought of as breaking rocks into dirt. Then, the small intestine carries the nutrients along until they are absorbed into the bloodstream. With whole foods, this absorption might take six to eight hours. But today's processed foods are often high in fructose, and fructose can be absorbed in as little as sixty to ninety minutes. The problem with fast absorption is that your body has to do a hormonal juggling act to manage your blood sugar levels. This pushes you into survival mode.

Fructose has several direct effects on belly fat, as well. When your fat is exposed to fructose, it causes your adrenals to make more stress hormones.[7] The adrenal glands make a strong stress hormone called *cortisol* and a weak stress hormone called *cortisone*. Fructose literally causes your fat to take the weak stress hormone and make it into the stronger one.[8] Finally, the fructose leaves your blood sugar so unstable that you end up making extra cortisol for hours in an attempt to fix the situation.[9]

liz's story, a study of food intolerances

Liz is a dramatic example of how much a sensitivity to certain foods can slow weight loss. At 45, she had been struggling with her weight for over a decade. It crept up in the years after her second child was born, and seemed unwilling to budge. She tried a low-fat diet when they were popular and just ended up gaining weight. Out of desperation, she even tried HCG hormone injections along with a 500-calorie-per-day diet. With this regimen she was able to lose 20 pounds, but then she gained back 26 in the months that followed.

Liz found the concept of carbohydrate cycling intuitive and easy to learn, but she did not want to avoid some of the dietary triggers. She came to see me after a month on the Adrenal Reset Diet, while still eating bread and cheese. She and her kids had a routine of serving bread with their meals and sprinkling cheese pretty heavily on their vegetables. In four weeks she had managed to lose 3 pounds, but she was frustrated that the weight was not coming off faster. I told her to try for the next four weeks to do things just as she had, but to change her evening bread to rice and change the veggies with cheese to veggies dipped in hummus.

During the next four weeks she was happy to see her weight come down by over 8 pounds. What really surprised her was the fact that she could breathe through her nose at night for the first time in a very long time. I explained to her how dietary intolerances can make airborne allergies worse, and that it is common to see symptoms like nasal congestion improve when reactive foods are avoided.

To learn more about which foods may be holding your health hostage, take the quiz from JJ Virgin, author of *The Virgin Diet,* at www.adrenalresetdiet.com/resources.

toxic proteins

Foods today contain higher amounts of toxic proteins, which can trigger survival mode. Because of this, the rates of dangerous allergies to foods like peanuts or shellfish have gone up many-fold during the last few decades. Most experts believe that food allergies are more common today because our foods are higher in chemicals and are different in many ways from how they were in the past.

An increase can also be seen in milder food reactions; these are often less obvious than allergies, what we call *intolerances*. Celiac disease is an example of a delayed food intolerance. They are most common in regard to wheat, dairy, and eggs. These foods contain large amounts of complex proteins that can be hard to digest, and reactions to these foods can cause many ongoing symptoms and can directly contribute to weight gain.

The protein in dairy is called *casein*, while wheat contains *gluten* and eggs contain *albumin*. The problem with these proteins is that they can trigger immune reactions, even when they do not cause obvious immediate symptoms, like pain or bloating.[10, 11]

A food allergy or intolerance presents a situation in which your immune cells attack something they deem to be dangerous. Even if those cells are wrong, the attack process increases inflammation dramatically, signaling your body to go into survival mode, and the fuel switch to go to "fat" mode.[12, 13]

As we discuss particular causes of bodily stress, it is good to bear in mind that there can be substantial overlap in the causes. Why do we react to toxic proteins more today than in the past? The processing of foods and the ever-increasing burden of environmental toxins both change our intestinal flora. Processed carbohydrates and the daily onslaught of toxicants from our air, water, and homes can damage the bacteria that assist in breaking down our proteins. When proteins aren't broken down properly, or are less digested, they are more apt to trigger immune responses.

Food intolerances have also been shown to trigger anxiety, which raises stress levels.[14] And once those reactive foods start raising your stress load, you become even more vulnerable to their effects. This sets in play a vicious cycle of food reactions causing stress, and stress making food reactions worse, until your body goes into survival mode and you gain weight.[15] Other problems that result from these reactions include gas and bloating, joint pain, and skin rashes.

The Adrenal Reset Diet focuses on high-quality nontoxic proteins from vegetables, nuts, seeds, beans, seafood, poultry, and lean meat.

trigger #2: environmental pollutants

Along with our increased consumption of processed foods, the numerous pollutants we are exposed to daily can trigger our bodies to go into survival mode. They do this by chemically activating the storage enzymes of the liver. These environmental pollutants can be found in our air and water, leached from the containers out of which we eat, and even emitted by artificial light.

a chemical soup

Sometimes pregnant women notice that their babies kick and move the most when poor mom is trying to get some sleep. It may seem odd, but your liver is also most active at night. The body's ability to detoxify depends on the cycle that our liver goes through each day. So, the liver does its best work cleaning out your body during your deep sleep. This is also when your liver is able to convert your food into energy for your muscles. When the body is full of pollutants, though, your liver never gets to rest and it ends up sending both calories and toxins to your belly fat instead.

How much are we exposed to environmental pollutants? Since 1900, over 3 million synthetic chemicals have been released into the world. Each day we eat and breathe in thousands of them without knowing it. This toxic exposure is now regarded as one of the more significant factors in the modern obesity epidemic. Many of these chemicals are formally categorized as *obesogens*, meaning that they are known to cause obesity, even in those who are not overeating.

The increase in the number of chemicals we are exposed to daily and the amount of that exposure both coincide with the onset of population-wide weight gain. A variety of chemicals have been shown to cause this weight gain, even with exposure at levels far below those that would cause apparent symptoms and that are well within the range of what we commonly experience. Key toxins include heavy metals such as lead or mercury, solvents, pesticides, and plastic by-products.

These chemicals are known to hurt the adrenal glands and change how our genes work. Because of their genetic effects, they can cause weight gain in those who are exposed to them, as well as later in their children and grandchildren. Many of these chemicals build up in our fat tissue, and since they are hard to process, they keep the fat locked in place and are seemingly impossible to get rid of.

plastic by-products

One substance that is shown to cause weight gain is a plastic by-product called Bisphenol A (BPA). BPA is present in many of our foods, as well as in our air and water. It enters our food as a by-product of packaging and as a contaminant from ground water. In a UK study from 2012, fat samples were taken from a group of seventeen people who had abdominal surgeries, and they were analyzed for levels of BPA. Significant levels were found to be present in every person studied; the more BPA was present, the more the participant's fat cells showed signs of fast growth. Although this was worse with higher amounts of BPA, even those with the lowest measurable amounts had unusual fat-cell growth. The conclusion was that their fat cells were changing the weaker stress hormones into stronger stress hormones.[16]

Along with making fat cells more aggressive, common toxic substances have been shown to raise the severity of our response to everyday stressors. Environmental lead has been causing human suffering from the earliest days of metal production to the present day. Most of our current exposure to lead is leftover remnants from lead-fortified gasoline and lead-based paint. A study from 2007 showed that those with the highest amounts of lead in their bodies produced the highest amounts of cortisol in response to routine stressors.[17]

light pollution

Environmental pollutants hurt cortisol cycles, which in addition to leading to fat deposition also disrupt sleep patterns. Sleep is likewise strained as a result of light pollution—the combination of exposure to artificial light and the lack of exposure to sunlight. Our ability to control our weight depends on deep sleep, which is directed by cues from the sun. Each new study strengthens the evidence for the connection between weight and sleep. In the last five years alone, over 270 research projects have evaluated how sleep affects body weight. Some of the newer results are giving us clues as to how exactly sleep regulates fat deposits. Once again, the adrenal glands are central to the story.

In a state of healthy sleep, the cortisol levels are reduced to their lowest levels of the day. This break from cortisol allows calories to be made into energy for our muscles. If cortisol is not able to shut down all the way, those same calories end up creating fat; and along with the fat being over-fed, the muscle tissue gets starved. This is the dilemma of adrenal dysfunction: too much fuel is present in the form of fat, but too little fuel is available to the muscles in the form of glycogen. This starts the vicious cycle of weight gain and fatigue, and it moves the body from thriving to just surviving.

Sleep is critical to so many of our body's functions, but is also an explanation for why many diets just can't work. It's clear that if your sleep is disrupted, your waistline will pay for it. But how does this happen? First, it is good to realize that sleep happens only when cortisol levels are low. Throughout the day, healthy people make a burst of cortisol to wake up and then it shuts off when they go to sleep. If your blood sugar level gets too low, your body will have to make more cortisol to raise it. If someone develops low blood sugar later in the day, he or she can end up with elevated nighttime cortisol levels and poor sleep quality. This is a problem with low-carbohydrate diets. In one such study, a group of healthy, lean men with no sleep problems were put on low-carbohydrate diets and their sleep quality was closely monitored. In as little as 48 hours, the time it took for them to fall asleep, how deeply they stayed asleep, and how much quality REM sleep they had decreased.[18]

The Adrenal Reset Diet is the first diet that carefully times carbohydrate consumption to ensure quality sleep and low nighttime cortisol levels.

trigger #3: the pressures of modern life

Life today brings with it change and uncertainty. Even though our lives are rarely in danger, our days are filled with constant low-level stressors that take the form of text messages, emails, deadlines, and distractions. We also face more frequent major stressors like job relocations and frequent separations from our extended families. Some estimates show that the pressures of modern life may have risen by as much as 30 percent just since the 1980s.[19]

Pressure is real and we all feel it, but can it directly cause weight gain? This was the question asked in a study of 54,000 women who were tracked over fifteen years. At several points during the study, the researchers measured the participants' body weight and used questionnaires to determine their total stress load. The data consistently showed that those with the highest stress loads gained the most weight.[20]

A related study has proven that pressure changes our appetite. In a group of women aged 40 to early 50s, stress levels were compared to food choices. Specifically, the women were asked to prepare a presentation for a job interview while a panel of "judges" observed. In the first stage of the experiment, the women were given a paper and pen, and were told that they would have five minutes to prepare notes for the presentation. The notes were taken away, and the "judges" watched the presentations without any signs of approval, like smiles or nods. Then, the participants were asked to do hard mental arithmetic while the judges scolded them for working too slowly. When the experiment was over, the participants were first tested for their cortisol levels and then invited to a buffet, not knowing that what they ate was being monitored. Those with the greatest cortisol disruption were the ones who ate the most chocolate cake and the least amount of vegetables.[21]

Another study proved the same phenomenon in a group of 333 high school students in Korea. The students were given questionnaires to determine how much pressure they felt in school, and then they were ranked into low-, medium-, and high-pressure groups. Those who felt under more pressure consistently ate larger meals and more frequently ate high-sugar foods, such as sodas, pastries, candies, chocolates, breads, and sweetened milk.[22]

Some have linked obesity to the addictive nature of today's foods and their high levels of sugar, fat, and salt. Although toxic food is definitely a factor in weight gain, brain scientists have shown that we are susceptible to food-based addictions only when we are in a higher state of pressure.[23]

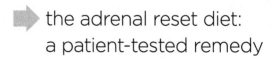

the adrenal reset diet: a patient-tested remedy

Once you see how dietary, mental, and physical/environmental triggers lead to weight gain, it becomes apparent why dieting generally fails. Eating less than you are used to eating and exercising more than you normally do only heighten mental stress. Working with, rather than against, your body's stress management system is the key to successful weight loss.

The Adrenal Reset Diet (ARD) is carefully engineered to address the major triggers of weight gain. Carbohydrates are cycled throughout the day, with most consumed in the evening. This lowers nighttime cortisol production and reverses the effects processed foods have on your visceral fat (see Table 1.2). Circadian repair is accomplished through detoxification and the therapeutic use of light to undo the effects pollution has had on your liver. Clearing your

TABLE 1.2. OVERVIEW OF THE ADRENAL RESET DIET

PROBLEMS	PROCESSED FOOD	POLLUTANTS	PRESSURES OF LIFE
Details	Fructose Toxic proteins	Environmental Light	Relationships Work Finances
Consequences	Adrenal Fat Switch gets set to survival mode. Hunger increases, energy decreases, and food is stored as fat.		

mind through simple breathing exercises helps reduce the effects of life's pressures on your brain.

By gaining a better understanding of your adrenal glands and their function in the next chapter, you will find that lasting weight loss is as simple as an adrenal reset.

your adrenals and how they control your weight

CHAPTER 1 DISCUSSED HOW STRESS HURTS THE ADRENALS AND can be a big part of weight gain. But what exactly are your adrenal glands and how can they help you get slim?

The adrenal glands are a couple of little lumps of tissue that sit on top of your kidneys, deep inside your lower back. They are spongy, orange, and shaped like little pyramids. Each one is about the size of a sugar cube and about the weight of three or four paperclips.[1]

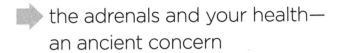

the adrenals and your health— an ancient concern

The view of the adrenal glands as having vast control over our health is hardly a new concept. Many ancient cultures believed that the adrenal glands contain some magic substance that allows life to exist and disappears when we die. It seemed intuitive to many ancient cultures that life is the product of an unseen, magical force, and that we are born with a supply of this force. The healthier our parents are, the more of the force we start out with. The quicker we use it up, the faster we age.

An Ayurvedic medical text dating back to roughly 100 BCE referred to that force as *Ojas*. It was said that Ojas was responsible for strength, health, and longevity. Chinese medicine has a similar

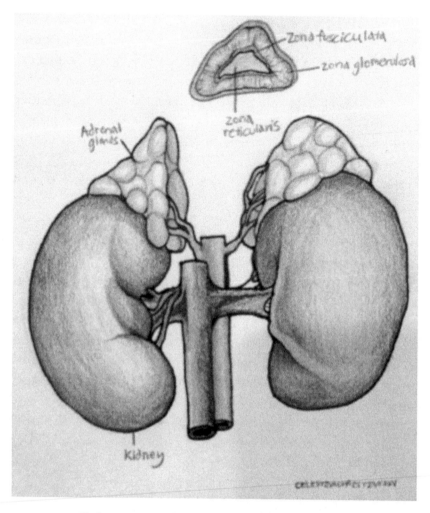

concept, called *Jing*. It is thought that Jing is the source of health and vitality. We are said to have a limited supply of Jing at birth, and that herbs, meditation, and breathing exercises are able to add to it. The inevitable process of aging is from the loss of our Jing, and it is said that it is used up more quickly by overwork and lack of sleep.

This is similar to our modern concept of aging, speeded up by today's high stress. The Chinese felt the Jing resided, not somewhere obvious like the heart or in the head, but just above the kidneys, where we now know the adrenal glands are. (They also felt the Jing was vulnerable to the effects of cold. That's why many Chinese traditional garments had layers of padding sewn in over the kidneys to keep the area warm and protect the Jing.)

In the 1930s, Dr. Weston A. Price traveled the world to study the health of pre-modern people. Pioneers in the early years of North American exploration often suffered from scurvy, a disease that develops from a lack of vitamin C, as was the case over long winters with no fresh fruits or vegetables. Dr. Price discovered that Native Americans had some awareness of the power of the adrenal glands. They ate the adrenal glands of game animals as a special strengthening food long before modern science knew what these glands were. Furthermore, the Alaskan Inuit and the lower states' Native Americans did not seem to get scurvy, a condition that develops from lack of vitamin C, though they had long winters when no fruits or vegetable were available. When Dr. Price asked about this, the Native Americans dismissed him by saying that only white men got scurvy. Later, an elder confided a secret: during the winter it was tradition that, after killing a large animal, the fatty tissue above the kidneys be divided among the tribe and eaten promptly. Although it was not known to Dr. Price then, the adrenal glands have high concentrations of vitamin C and would have helped ward off scurvy. We now know that vitamin C is also needed for good adrenal function in humans.

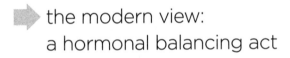

the modern view: a hormonal balancing act

Today we know that the adrenal glands are critical parts of the endocrine system, which is the group of glands that produce the body's hormones. Nearly every facet of good health is a product of the delicate balance of these hormones. For example, your hormone levels determine the answers to questions like:

- Are you in a good mood?
- How well do you sleep at night?
- Is it easy to maintain your weight?
- Do you get afternoon crashes?
- Is your blood sugar steady or are you diabetic?
- Do you heal promptly after injuries?

getting down to business: the endocrine system

The endocrine system is so powerful that it needs checks and balances to operate properly. You can think of it like a corporation. Imagine you have a CEO who has the highest level of responsibility; this would be your *hypothalamus*. Living deep inside your brain and no larger than a pearl, it runs the whole show. Below the CEO is a manager, who communicates to the workers; this would be the *pituitary gland*. Nestled next to your hypothalamus, and no bigger than a pea, it keeps track of the workers. Then you have the team who carries out all these orders; along with the adrenals, they consist of the *pineal gland*, the *thyroid*, the *pancreas*, and the *testicles* or *ovaries*. These glands release hormones that are carried in the bloodstream and work throughout the body to control essential chemical functions. These functions include:

- Pineal gland: regulates sleep cycles

- Thyroid: controls energy production

- Ovaries: produces reproductive hormones and does tissue repair

- Testicles: produces reproductive hormones and does tissue repair

- Pancreas: regulates blood sugar

the busy life of your adrenals

The adrenal glands have three layers nestled inside each other, like the layers of an onion. Each layer's job is unique, so some researchers believe it may be more accurate to think of each of them as three glands rather than one.

The outer layer's main job is the regulation of salts (electrolytes) in the blood, the blood pressure, and the body's acid levels. The middle layer primarily controls blood sugar, but it is also in charge of the stress response (inflammation) and controls how cells use the hormones from the other glands. The inner layer, working in conjunction with the ovaries or testicles, makes the sex hormones used in reproduction, such as estrogen or testosterone. The inner layer also helps with tissue repair and immune function.

Your adrenal glands control a staggering list of vital functions in your body. The biggest ones are:

- Regulation of other hormones

- Balance of electrolytes

- When to turn off inflammation

- Fight-or-flight response

- Sleep and waking cycles

- Blood sugar

- Body weight

Have you heard about the latest research on multitasking? Basically, it does not work. The more tasks we try to do at the same time, the worse we do any of them. The same rule applies to your adrenal glands. The more demands that are placed on them at one time, the more apt they are to move into survival mode. As you will see, once this happens, weight gain becomes more likely. Later in the book I give you diet and lifestyle methods that can gently remove this stress load. For now, though, it is important to understand how the adrenals can easily get too much put on their metaphorical plate—and why that overload changes how your fat responds to what is on that plate. So, let's first look a bit closer at all the adrenal functions.

hormone regulation

The adrenals have an important job that is not shared by any other glands. They keep your system working well by regulating how the other hormones get used. That is, once a hormone has been released, it has to be absorbed into a cell before it can do anything. Whether or not the cell absorbs that hormone is determined by how much cortisol is in the bloodstream at that moment.

cortisol control

Correct hormone levels are so vital to your health that they require many means of regulation. The hypothalamus and the pituitary gland are in the brain, and they control how much hormone is released from the various glands.

Once the hormones are released, the adrenal glands make the decision on how much should be used. This system works because each of the body's cells has a wall around it that governs what gets in and what gets out. Hormones only work when a door in the wall opens and lets them get inside the cell. Cortisol from the adrenal glands opens that door to let the hormone into the cell. When cortisol is not present, the door remains closed and the hormone stays outside the cell.

What this means is that, even if the other glands are doing their jobs perfectly, it may seem like they are not working correctly if the adrenals don't let their hormones into the cells. For example, if your adrenals are not working properly, you may have symptoms of low thyroid, such as fatigue or weight gain. And this can happen even if your thyroid is perfectly healthy, because your cells are not using those thyroid hormones. Thus, adrenal dysfunction can lead to fatigue, weight gain, and depression, just as thyroid disease can. Because the adrenals work to help the thyroid, people who experience problems with one gland may actually have problems with the other.

electrolytes

At a fundamental level, our bodies work like storage batteries. We have an electric charge, and reactions occur when this charge moves from one place to another inside the body's fluids. Yet these charges move only when the balance of minerals in the fluids is correct. These minerals are called *electrolytes*, and they include sodium, potassium, chloride, calcium, and magnesium. Adrenal hormones like aldosterone work to make sure that the levels of these electrolytes are neither too high nor too low—that they are just right for good health. When they are not right, the muscles cramp and ache, digestion works poorly, and the brain cannot think clearly.

inflammation

When you bump your knee, it hurts. If you bump it hard enough, it will also swell. It may look reddened and be warm to the touch. And if you bump it really hard, it might be difficult to move at first. These symptoms are all signs of inflammation: pain, swelling, redness, heat, poor function. The word *inflammation* is derived from the Latin *inflammo*, meaning "to set on fire." For over a century, researchers have known that nearly every disease is related to excessive inflammation.

Inflammation can be caused by quick and obvious factors, like a bump on the knee. It can also be caused by slow and hidden factors, like infections, nutrient deficiencies, or stress. Despite all the bad things that come from too much inflammation, some inflammation is good. In the case of acute trauma or hard exercise, inflammation helps us heal. When it works right, this healing occurs in three stages.

In the first stage, the blood vessels get leaky. They become like a soaker hose used in the garden, the type that lets water drip through its lining. This allows nutrients and immune cells to move outside of the blood vessels to the cells where they are needed. In the second stage, immune cells digest debris and clean the damaged tissue. In the third stage, the immune cells help start the process of tissue repair. However, sometimes problems occur. For example, this inflammatory response can go on too long or can start when it is not needed. It's this "unneeded" inflammation that is thought to be the source of most chronic disease. The more inflammation we have, the shorter we will live and the worse we will feel.

When the adrenal glands are working properly, they can shut off the inflammation as soon as its work is done. But when your adrenal function is not at its best, that inflammation is poorly controlled, and this can manifest as chronic pain. For instance, you could start with a minor overuse injury like tennis elbow, but if the adrenals do not regulate the inflammation as they should, the repair may not be completed and the pain may become ongoing.

sleeping and waking cycles

What time you wake up and what time you feel sleepy are events carefully controlled by your adrenal glands. This timing is called your *circadian rhythm*. Your adrenals have a partner in this job, the pineal gland; it is one of the glands in your brain, and it makes a hormone important for sleep, called *melatonin*. The pineal gland is extremely sensitive to how much light your eyes take in, the exact wavelengths of that light, and even whether the light enters your eyes from above you or below you. It seems we are better adapted to sunlight from above us than to TV light from in front of us.

You could imagine cortisol and melatonin as two hormones on a seesaw. When you wake in the morning on your own, it is from a surge of cortisol that was released about an hour earlier. This release is like an internal coffeemaker that is timed to be ready when you're up and about. When the cortisol surges, the melatonin production is stopped. For an illustration of this relationship, see opposite.

In the evening, when you get tired, there's been a surge of melatonin that was started about twenty minutes earlier. The cortisol production starts being lowered after lunchtime and is almost completely shut off by bedtime, when you are healthy and thriving. This allows the melatonin to take over. Many people who have adrenal dysfunction lack this proper fluctuation of cortisol. They may not make a nice morning surge or it may not shut off adequately while sleeping.

The Cortisol/Melatonin Cycle

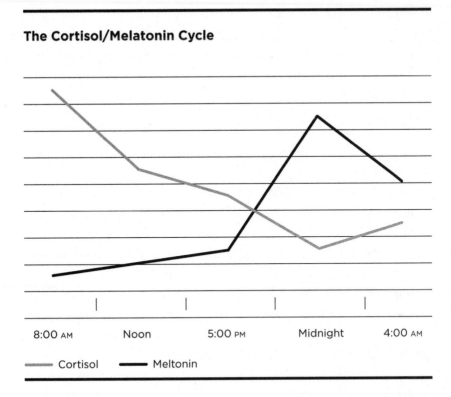

| 8:00 AM | Noon | 5:00 PM | Midnight | 4:00 AM |

Cortisol　　Meltonin

blood sugar

Along with all these other jobs, the adrenal glands regulate blood sugar. Here, the pancreas is their closest ally. When you have not eaten for a few hours, your adrenals release cortisol. This moves carbohydrates out of their stores in your muscle and liver and into your bloodstream to keep your brain fed. When you are thriving, this can happen mostly through the efforts of the pancreas, with little work from your adrenals.

But if your blood sugar drops off suddenly, your adrenal glands have to work harder and make extra cortisol. This happens when you miss a meal, eat too few good carbs, or eat too many bad carbs. These elevated cortisol levels may make you feel stressed out or edgy when you're hungry. A drop in blood sugar triggers the same fight-or-flight response that fear does. In summary, when your blood sugar is well controlled, you feel energized and you stay lean.

When your blood sugar is poorly controlled, you feel depressed and you gain weight. And when the latter situation goes on for long periods of time, bad things happen, like diabetes, heart disease, and cancer.

the survival mode

Although they have several jobs, the adrenals are likely best known for their role in regulating the body's survival mode. When you are faced with a stressful situation, the adrenals produce hormones that allow the body to divert energy away from day-to-day maintenance and put it all toward getting you through the task at hand.

To understand survival mode and how it ties in to body weight, it helps to understand its history. For the past 200,000 years, the human genes have been adapting to survival challenges. There were times when early humans needed to act much faster than the speed of thought. This required them to push their bodies harder than generally possible for brief, decisive moments.

In the face of immediate danger, they ran or fought, and they did so harder than they normally could. This response was triggered by the adrenal glands through their release of stress hormones. Since one of these chemicals was first discovered in the adrenal glands, it was named *adrenalin*. When early humans survived the danger, the fight-or-flight response ended; pleasurable *endorphins* were then released as further incentive for surviving another day.

Today the word *adrenalin* makes many think of "adrenaline junkies," those who become addicted to the rush that accompanies dangerous situations. Ironically, it is not the adrenalin at all that they are addicted to but, rather, the endorphin release that comes after surviving a dangerous situation. Unfortunately, unless the danger is real or at least perceived to be, the endorphin rush will not arrive.

chronic stress and your adrenals

When faced with high levels of the stress that comes from your consuming processed food, exposure to pollution, or the pressures of life, the adrenal glands have to work harder. If they are pushed too hard, it's as if they flip a switch inside your body that stays on survival mode. When the switch is off, your body is thriving and it adjusts your metabolism to keep your weight steady, even if you change your diet or exercise routines. But when it's in survival mode, your body holds on to every available calorie and converts it to visceral fat. In the past when humans faced famine, survival mode was helpful. Today, we get triggered into survival mode by many things that are not really immediate dangers. Thus, what used to help us survive is now the cause of our greatest threat. If you think this is an overstatement, keep reading.

is stress really such a big deal?

How much can stress affect our health? Over the last several decades, a few situations have come together that allow us to get a glimpse at how much some factors affect our health compared to other factors. One of the most dramatic involved people affected by the 1986 nuclear disaster at Chernobyl.

The very name Chernobyl conjures up images of widespread disaster and contamination. A nuclear reactor broke down releasing 400 times as much radiation as the atomic bomb had in Hiroshima. Many have called it the worst man-made disaster in human history. Over 200,000 people were forcibly relocated for their safety. Radiation at those levels damages human bodies at a molecular level. The very DNA inside every cell can become altered, leading to pain, disease, and suffering.

But being forced to leave your community, livelihood, and ancestral homeland is also a trauma. Immediate consequences include posttraumatic stress syndrome, as well as anxiety and depression. Long term, this heightened level of stress changes food preferences, tendencies toward addiction, and also self-care.

The 30 square kilometers around Chernobyl are an official "dead zone" into which access is minimal and strictly controlled. Yet many chose to return. They decided that separation from home was more of a trauma than invisible radiation. Most were already adults at the time of the accident, and hence their numbers are steadily dwindling. Comparisons have been made between the lives of the Chernobyl "settlers" and those of the Chernobyl evacuees who did not return. The settlers suffer symptoms on a daily basis from the radiation they live with, and their health has clearly been affected. Yet the trauma of being a refugee may be even greater; as short as the life spans of the Chernobyl settlers is, that of the refugees is ten years shorter yet.[2]

Can stress really change our health in measurable ways? Is it really a powerful enough factor to cause tangible consequences, like weight gain or disease? Clearly the answer is yes when you consider that the physical effects from Chernobyl may be less than the physical effects of psychological stress.

how the adrenals control weight

Now that you know about the main jobs of your adrenal glands, let's talk about one more job that may be the most important for you now: how they control your weight.

People who have high amounts of cortisol in their bodies from adrenal diseases or from medications like prednisone gain lots of belly fat regardless of their diet or activity. Scientists realized this as far back as the 1950s, and in consequence many wondered if adrenal hormones could cause obesity. To test this, they measured levels of hormones like cortisol in the bloodstream of people of different weights. The results were not clear; some heavy people had more cortisol and others had less. This caused the research to be dropped for many decades.

In the last few years, though, we have learned that adrenal hormones are not just made by the adrenal glands but also by visceral fat, the liver, and the brain.[3] Newer studies are showing that when you measure how much cortisol is in the whole body, versus just what's in the blood, the heavier people clearly do have more of it.[4] The reason for this is a group of enzymes that I call the Adrenal Fat Switch (AFS). Their names are *c-jun-n terminal kinase, insulin protease,* and *11-betahydroxysteroid dehydrogenase.* When we go into survival mode, these enzymes make adrenal hormones increase our fat storage. You can think of the fat switch as a stress amplifier. Weight loss cannot occur if this switch is turned on and you are in survival mode.

The Adrenal Reset Diet repairs the adrenal rhythms that let us shut off the fat switch and lose weight.

Researchers used to think that the timing of the AFS enzymes was not possible to change. However, exciting recent data have shown that both the amount of cortisol made by the adrenals and the activity of the fat switch are changeable by simple food choices.[5] That is, the right foods at the right times can reset the whole adrenal system, including the fat switch.

The AFS Cycle

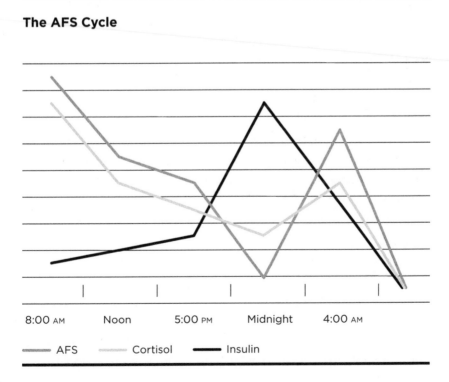

| 8:00 AM | Noon | 5:00 PM | Midnight | 4:00 AM |

AFS   Cortisol   Insulin

how food affects your rhythms

How does this adrenal system work? It turns out that higher amounts of protein and fat in your diet cause more cortisol to be released, which turns off the fat switch. This is good for the morning rhythm. Higher carbohydrate meals decrease cortisol release, and they turn on the fat switch. When you are thriving, thus, the fat switch is set on "off." This helps you burn calories and use the food to make energy for the following day. The Adrenal Reset Diet is the first program to utilize diet to correct these fat-switch rhythms.

 # why dieting is a disaster

What does typical dieting do? By reducing the number of calories or carbohydrates consumed, you actually increase the activity of the AFS, making regaining weight happen more easily.[6] This is the same mechanism as occurs under stress. The more stressors you face, the more your adrenal system becomes disrupted and the more apt you are to have your switch flipped into survival mode.

the cycle of weight gain

Given the role the adrenal glands play in regulating stress response and the number of things that disrupt their action, it is easy to see how dysfunctional weight gain can become a vicious cycle; see the illustration that follows.

Here is how it plays out:

- Stress comes from depression, work, relationships, dieting, toxins.

- Stress leads to dysfunction of the adrenal glands, raising cortisol levels.

- Increased cortisol levels cause you to store abdominal fat.

- The abdominal fat makes you crave sugar, fat, and salt.

- The abdominal fat makes even more cortisol by itself.

- There's poor energy production because fuel is being stored instead of burned, leading to fatigue.

- Fatigue and health changes create depression.

- Depression causes more stress.

Cycle of Weight Gain

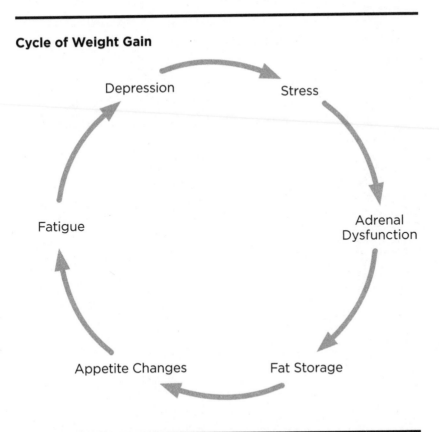

stress study: karen's story

Karen was a psychologist who focused her work on marriage and family therapy. After hearing great feedback about her, I started referring patients to her. For years, though I knew she was a good resource for others, I had not met her in person. One day she came in to see me about her own health. After being naturally thin most of her life, she found maintaining her weight had become a major struggle in the last several years. Having seen many of our mutual patients lose weight, she decided to see me herself.

Karen mentioned going to the gym several times per week, even though she never used to. She was also trying to eat regular meals and avoid junk food, but her weight kept going up. As a routine screen for her level of stress, we checked her daily cortisol rhythm. Karen's showed a high state of chronic stress and no nighttime cortisol decrease. When I asked her about this, she broke down in tears. Despite being a marriage expert, her own marriage was on the rocks. When she was not at home struggling with her relationship, she was with her clients, feeling like an imposter.

I helped Karen with a six-week Adrenal Reset Diet menu and gave her some specific breathing exercises to lower her cortisol levels. I also encouraged her to seek professional help to aid her in coping with her failing relationship. By the end of the six weeks, she was down over 20 pounds and feeling hopeful about her health and her life.

➡ reset your adrenals and reset your weight

Weight gain is *not* a matter of too much fuel coming in and too little fuel going out. When in good health, we are able to keep our weight at a range conducive to our good health despite inevitable variations in day-to-day food intake. Circadian hormones regulate our weight. In survival mode, these hormones act to allow as much weight gain and quick energy release as possible. Thus, weight gain is the product of these hormones being stuck in survival mode. Being stuck in survival mode changes both what happens to the food we eat and which foods we prefer to eat.

As mentioned earlier, your adrenals have many aspects of your health to keep in check. These include regulating your other hormones, controlling inflammation, the fight-or-flight response, sleep and waking cycles, and your blood sugar. They also are controlling your weight. The more work they have to do for any of these jobs, the more apt they are to put you in storage mode, where you gain weight.

By cycling carbohydrates—eating them at the right time each day—cortisol can be brought back to a healthy rhythm, with high levels of cortisol in the morning and low levels at night. This fixes the fat switch to "off" and causes calories to move into the muscles, which produces energy, instead of moving them into the visceral fat, which makes you sluggish and causes weight gain.

The Adrenal Reset Diet is the first diet that is structured to reset your Adrenal Fat Switch, which leads to lasting fat loss. Next up, how it works.

how the
reset works

ending the protein
vs. carbs debate

NUTRITION WAS SO SIMPLE IN THE LATE 1980S. WE BELIEVED that dietary fat caused fat on our bodies and fat in our blood vessels. It seemed so logical. First, low fat was in vogue, but the inevitable extension of this was the fat-free movement. If fat was bad, then fat-free was good. I worked in a health food store at the time, and one evening a group of my coworkers met up at one of their homes. Our host was a bright athletic woman who greeted us with bowls of jelly beans and pretzels. She asked us, "Isn't it amazing how good fat-free snacks can be?" I remember thinking that even though these foods were fat-free, they still were not healthy.

Soon afterward, the heretical notion of "healthy fats" became public and we realized that not all fats are bad. We can look back on these ideas and laugh, but today many have swung to another extreme with the idea that carbs are the sole villain. In some nutritional circles, bacon has become the new jelly bean. Just like there are good fats, you will learn that there are also good carbs and good times for carbs.

One way or another, nearly all of the major diets since the dawn of the obesity crisis have been focused on carbs. Low-carb diets say that we need to eat fewer carbs and more protein. Higher-carb diets say protein and fat should be avoided and that carbs are good.

Credible scientists, physicians, and dieticians have lined up on both sides of this argument. They agree that processed carbs are bad news, but they have opposite views on foods like beans, brown rice, sweet potatoes, and low-sugar fruit.

Which side is right? You'll soon learn that the answer depends on the time of day.

carbs—can't live with 'em, can't live without 'em

Carbohydrates are one of the main macronutrients in our diets, *macro* meaning "big." These are nutrients that we consume in amounts large enough to see, as opposed to the invisible *micro*-nutrients like vitamins and minerals. When you look at a chicken breast, you're seeing long chains of protein. When you see a bowl of rice, you are looking at thousands of strands of carbohydrate. Along with protein and carbohydrate, the remaining macronutrient is fat.

Perhaps the biggest source of controversy and confusion in the world of nutrition is the carbohydrate. High-carb and low-carb advocates have been arguing back and forth for over a century now. Long before the Atkins diet, William Banting's 1863 pamphlet "Letter on Corpulence [obesity], Addressed to the Public" is considered by many to be the first low-carb diet book.

Carbohydrates are normally the main source of sugar in the bloodstream. There is no debate that reactions involving unstable blood sugar are present in obesity, as well as in many chronic diseases including diabetes, some cancers, heart disease, and Alzheimer's disease.

If carbs form blood sugar, and abnormal blood sugar levels cause so many problems, why not just give them up? Many in the more strict versions of the Paleo movement encourage just that—the avoidance of all fruit, grains, and starchy vegetables. On the surface this might seem logical, but so many things in the body do not work the way you would expect.

low carbs raise cortisol

One problem is that when you cut your carbs too much, cortisol rises. Remember that one of cortisol's jobs is keeping your blood sugar up. There's a drop in blood sugar when you miss meals or you are fasting, but it also happens if your meals are too low in carbs. Your body needs cortisol to take glucose from your muscles and liver. This rise in cortisol can turn on the fat-storage enzymes and lead to poorer-quality sleep, both of which work against lasting weight loss.

low carbs can raise blood sugar

In treating people with diabetes, I use a tool called a *continuous glucose meter*. This meter allows me to monitor someone's blood sugar levels 24 hours of the day, for several days in a row. One of my unexpected findings was that most people who eat fewer than 50 grams of carbohydrates per day end up with more glucose in their blood than those who eat more carbohydrates. This is true for both diabetics and nondiabetics.

If blood glucose comes from carbs, why would avoiding carbs raise blood glucose? Here is what happens. When you have a meal without any carbs, your blood sugar starts to drop. To prevent it from getting too low, your adrenal glands make extra cortisol, which pulls glucose out of your muscles and liver. This not only leaves you without energy, it also raises your glucose more than a meal with healthy carbs would. Erratic blood glucose levels also cause fat storage and sugar cravings.

low carbs lead to poor sleep

The more we learn about how critical sleep is for fat loss, the more we want to avoid anything that works against it. One study compared a low-carb diet to a diet with moderate amounts of carbs, with the goal of observing its effects on sleep. Both diets contained 2,400 calories and provided substantial and equal amounts of food. After just 48 hours, the low-carbohydrate diet caused the participants to take longer to fall asleep, to get less total sleep, and to get less restful sleep.[1]

high carbs are also not the answer

If low-carb diets cause problems, should we just go to high-carb diets? No, because high-carb diets cause fat growth and fatigue as well.

Remember how low-carb diets can cause the body to make too much sugar? Any time we get too much of something, we convert it to something else. It turns out that high-carb diets cause the liver to make dangerous fats called triglycerides, which raise the risk of heart disease.[2] Some of the triglycerides stay stuck in the liver, which can lead to fatty liver disease. The rest of these triglycerides circulate through our blood vessels, raising the risk of heart disease and causing visceral fat growth.

High-carb diets are also a problem because they cause fatigue. A study was done to see how well four groups of people could do mental tasks after having different types of breakfasts. The first group skipped breakfast completely. The second had a high-carb breakfast, the third ate mixed protein and carbs, and the fourth ate mostly protein. Participants were given mental tasks every hour for four hours. In the first hour, everyone did better than those who had not eaten. By the second hour, the high-carb group was doing the worst; those with a moderate protein intake and those with a high protein intake were doing equally well. After the third hour, the high-protein group won, hands down.[3]

If you want to be energetic and mentally sharp during the day, a high-protein breakfast is the key. It works well because you are allowing your cortisol to have its morning spike and your insulin to stay at its natural morning low. The same holds true and is critical for losing fat.

the right carbs at the right time

If high-carb and low-carb diets both have problems, obviously we need some carbs. Like Goldilocks, we need to get them just right:

we need the right types of carbs, not too much, not too little, and not too early in the day.

how i created the reset: the concept of carb cycling

Many years ago I realized that our daily adrenal rhythms are what make or break our health. When they are in harmony, we are thriving. When they are off, we are just surviving. The stresses of modern life can easily disrupt these rhythms. So I wondered: since low blood sugar leads to high cortisol, and high blood sugar leads to low cortisol, could carbohydrates be used to help reset cortisol?

As always, I was my own first test subject. Without disrupting my sleep to test, I measured my glucose levels every minute with a special patch that sent a signal to a glucose meter. I also measured my cortisol levels every four hours while awake by collecting salivary samples.

Cortisol testing deserves a bit of explanation, since no methods are perfect. Cortisol is made by the adrenal glands, but the belly fat, the liver, and the brain also make it. Blood tests show how much cortisol you make during the moment of the blood draw. This is not perfect, because just the process of having your blood drawn can change your cortisol levels. Also, the testing result is just a snapshot of how much cortisol your adrenals are making. Salivary tests are a bit better because they show how much cortisol you produce at different times of the day. But even they are not perfect because they do not reflect how much cortisol you make outside of your adrenals. Hair cortisol and urine collections for twenty-four consecutive hours can show how much total cortisol you make from the adrenals and most of what you make in the fat, liver, and brain, but here also they don't show how your day's levels can vary. When I was forming and testing these theories, I used all three tests: blood tests, salivary tests, and urine tests.

In my initial personal experiment, my cortisol was higher in the morning and low at night, as it should be. Then I measured for two more days while eating no protein from morning until 3 PM and no carbs after 3 PM. Not only were my cortisol levels reversed, but I could not sleep! Even though I was careful not to increase my calorie intake, I also gained a few pounds and had evening sugar cravings. My glucose levels moved outside of the ideal by the second day. However, a few days of eating low carbs in the morning and lower protein in the evening pulled me back to normal sleep and good glucose control.

The next step was to enlist help from my patients. I chose a few who had erratic blood sugar levels, stubborn weight problems, and poor cortisol rhythms. I let them know the experimental nature of the idea, and I asked if they would mind trying out a new diet that cycled carbohydrates. The initial results were great. People consistently reported easier weight loss, fewer starch cravings, better energy levels, and better depth of sleep. I also saw dramatic reductions in the blood sugar of those who were diabetic or pre-diabetic.

Since that time, studies other than mine have proven that carbs can adjust the daily cortisol rhythm, although I have not found other studies that have used this as the cornerstone of a weight-loss plan.[4]

Now that you have learned that the *timing* of carbs is important, let's look a little more at them in general, as well as at the other macronutrients, so you can easily construct a diet that helps you thrive.

becoming a carb mechanic

All the foods we get from plants have healthy carbs. Most vegetables, such as leafy greens, onions, mushrooms, sprouts, celery, and tomatoes, have carbs but only in tiny amounts. Starchy vegetables, like carrots, squash, turnips, and corn, have more carbs. The highest amounts of carbs are found in grains, beans, and fruits.

Foods made with processed sugar and flour have unhealthy carbs.

In the modern diet, specific foods high in unhealthy carbs include breads, cold cereals, crackers, pastries, juices, pancakes, waffles, French toast, syrups, tortillas, sodas, cookies, cakes, and candies. Surprisingly, dried fruits and fruit juices can also be a problem, even fresh-squeezed juices with the pulp.

fiber and fructose: the old good carb / bad carb routine

Fiber and fructose are key parts of carbs you need to be aware of. Understanding them and their role in your health helps you make the best choices.

Fiber is the part of carbohydrates that we cannot digest, and it turns out that it has major health benefits. Fiber helps us lose weight, it helps our bodies remove toxins, and it protects our immune system.[5] The three main types of fiber are soluble, insoluble, and resistant.

insoluble fiber

Insoluble fiber is the type that does not dissolve in water. This is what most people think about when you say "fiber." It helps the intestinal tract stay regular and stabilizes the body's blood sugar. The highest sources of insoluble fiber are whole grains, nuts, green vegetables, and the skins of root vegetables.

BEST SOURCES: Brown rice, quinoa, barley, buckwheat, almonds, broccoli, cabbage, carrots, and potatoes with the skin.

soluble fiber

Soluble fiber dissolves in water and feeds the healthy bacteria of the intestinal tract; it also lowers abdominal fat and reduces cholesterol. It has been shown to reduce heart disease, make the immune system stronger, and can lower the risk of developing some cancers.[6]

Foods such as legumes; some grains like buckwheat, brown rice, and quinoa; and berries and seeds are especially high in soluble fiber.

BEST SOURCES: Lentils, garbanzo beans (chickpeas), blackberries, flax seed, and gluten free rolled oats.

resistant fiber

Resistant fiber is the new kid on the block. It is a unique type of starch that is digested, but only many hours later and only by the good bacteria. Also known as *resistant starch*, this fiber contains calories, but the majority of its calories are not usable and therefore cannot cause weight gain. Resistant fiber is remarkable since it creates little or no insulin response, unlike any other carbohydrate. In fact, it can even produce less of an insulin response than many non-carbohydrate foods like meat, poultry, and eggs. For this reason, many of the low-carb breakfasts on the Adrenal Reset Diet include foods high in resistant fiber.

BEST SOURCES: Boiled potatoes, cannellini beans, navy beans, great northern beans, and unripe bananas.

resistant fiber for fat loss

In a study of sixteen obese men and women with insulin resistance, resistant fiber was tested to see if it could help move glucose into the muscles and away from the fat stores. After just eight weeks, it was shown that the resistant fiber decreased blood sugar, decreased insulin, and increased the ability of the muscles to utilize glucose by 65 percent. These results occurred without diet and exercise—only the addition of resistant fiber.[7]

fructose

If fiber were the healthiest part of carbs, fructose would be the unhealthiest. Fructose is a kind of sugar that can exclusively be processed by your liver. Since your liver can only do so much at once, too much fructose can clog it. If our only source of fructose were whole fruit, this would not likely be a problem. However, since we are so overloaded with fructose from our processed foods, we have become even more sensitive to it. It is such a problem today that many consider fructose the greatest of several factors behind the obesity epidemic.

FIBER / FRUCTOSE RATIO

Since fiber is good and fructose is bad, how good a carb is for us can be determined by considering how much fiber it has compared to its fructose (its F:F ratio). The more fiber and the less fructose a carb has, the healthier it is for us. Table 3.1 gives the ratios of fiber to fructose for several unprocessed carbs. Those trying to lose weight should focus on carbs with a score of 4 or greater. (Please note that low-starch vegetables on the unlimited foods lists do not have significant amounts of fructose and can still be eaten freely.)

From looking at Table 3.1, it becomes apparent that foods are consistent within their categories. In general, beans are the best; gluten-free intact whole grains and vegetables were next best; and fruits had lots of variation.

paleo principles—how do they fit with the ARD?

In the last several years, the Paleo diet movement has had many positive effects on our nutritional beliefs. From it, people have become more conscious of the value of fresh organic vegetables, the need for high-quality lean protein, and the importance of avoiding synthetic and processed foods. Many have gotten a stronger sense of the dangers of unhealthy carbs. People have also gained a better understanding of how many health problems stem from foods and food ingredients like dairy, gluten, soy, and sugar, even when the foods themselves do not cause obvious and immediate bad reactions.

TABLE 3.1. FIBER / FRUCTOSE RATIO (F:F)

FOOD (AVG. SERVING)	FIBER (GRAMS)	FRUCTOSE (GRAMS)	FIBER/ FRUCTOSE RATIO
Black beans (½ cup)	10	<0.5	20
Kidney beans (½ cup)	10	<0.5	20
Pinto beans (½ cup)	10	<0.5	20
Great northern beans (½ cup)	8	<0.5	16
Brown rice, cooked (½ cup)	6	<0.5	12
Quinoa, cooked (½ cup)	6	<0.5	12
Buckwheat groats, cooked (½ cup)	5	<0.5	10
Broccoli (½ cup)	4	.5	8
Potatoes, boiled (½ cup)	4	.5	8
Gluten-free old-fashioned rolled oats, raw (½ cup)	4	<0.5	8
Sweet potatoes, peeled and cooked (½ cup)	3	<0.5	6
Carrots, cooked (2 medium)	2	0.5	4
Corn kernels, cooked (½ cup)	5	1.5	3.33
Raspberries (½ cup)	5	2	2.5
Cauliflower, raw (1 cup)	3	1.5	2
Blackberries (½ cup)	5	3	1.66
Peaches, with peel (1 medium)	2	1.2	1.66
Tomatoes (1 medium)	1.5	1	1.5
Baked beans (½ cup)	8	6	1.33
Dried figs (6 medium)	20	17	1.17

FOOD (AVG. SERVING)	FIBER (GRAMS)	FRUCTOSE (GRAMS)	FIBER/ FRUCTOSE RATIO
Blueberries (½ cup)	4	4	1
Strawberries (½ cup)	1.5	1.5	1
Pineapple chunks (½ cup)	2	2	1
Nectarines, with peel (1 medium)	2	2	1
Dried dates (3 deglet noor)	3	3	1
Eggplant, cooked and peeled, (½ cup)	3	4	0.75
Onion, raw (¼ cup)	1	1.5	0.66
Kiwifruit (1)	2	3	0.66
Dried apricots (½ cup)	5	8	0.63
Pear, with peel (1 medium)	6	10	0.6
Cabbage, raw (1 cup)	1.8	3	0.6
Banana (1 medium)	3	6	.5
Grapefruit (½ cup)	2	4	.5
Plums (1 medium)	1	2	.5
Apple (1 medium)	4	11	0.36
Raisins (¼ cup)	3	11	.27
Honeydew melon, cubed (1 cup)	1	5	.2
Dried dates (3 medjool)	4	21	.19
Cherries (½ cup)	1	7	.14
Mango, raw, cubed (½ cup)	2	16	0.125
Grapes (1 cup)	1	12	.08

Some within the Paleo movement have argued that all beans, legumes, and even gluten-free grains should be avoided because they contain chemicals like phytic acid. The argument is that these compounds can rob the body of minerals and leave a person deficient in essential nutrients. In fact, phytic acid does bind with minerals, but it does so within the foods before you eat them. Therefore, it cannot take minerals out of your body that you have already absorbed. The main negative factor involving phytic acid is that it hampers the absorption of iron in the foods that contain phytic acid. This means that if your only source of iron is plants, as in eating beans and spinach, you may not absorb enough iron. But if your diet includes animal sources of iron, such as dark-meat poultry and red meat, you will absorb the iron just fine, even if you eat foods with phytic acid, such as beans, in the same meal.

Phytic acid is not only harmless but is actually helpful for the immune system and may lower the risks of colon cancer.[8] Foods with phytic acid are also the best sources of insoluble fiber, which is important for a healthy balance of intestinal bacteria. Furthermore, many foods that Paleo enthusiasts do not avoid still have substantial amounts of phytic acid, some even more than the forbidden grains and beans; these include nuts, seeds, potatoes, and sweet potatoes. Without including gluten-free grains and legumes in your diet, the only other substantial source of carbs is fruit. And if fruit were your prime carb, your diet would end up being far too high in fructose.

In summary, gluten-free grains, starchy vegetables, and legumes are an important part of a healthy diet and should not be avoided.

how many carbs should you eat?

Carbs should make up between 35 and 45 percent of your calories. To get this amount, most of your carbs should come from vegetables and they should make up about half the mass of your day's food. You do not need that much with each meal, but you do want that much over the course of the day.

In terms of grams, 75 to 90 grams per day is best for most adults who exercise under an hour per day. How much is this? You can think of it as 1½ cups of cooked brown rice, pinto beans, or sweet potato. If you go below 50 grams per day, you will get very tired and lose muscle. In a study of adults, it was shown that eating under 50 grams of carbs blocked thyroid hormones and caused a 44 percent increase in muscle wasting.[9]

The best carbs to eat are the ones that burn the most slowly, like black beans, brown rice, quinoa, or boiled potatoes. After you eat a meal, the carbohydrates are broken down in the stomach and absorbed into the bloodstream by the small intestines. When carbs are absorbed fast, they lead to a drop in blood sugar and an elevation in cortisol. Based on this cortisol response, the same carbs could be burned as fuel or stored as fat.

The types of carbs that get absorbed too fast come from foods that have been highly processed. These foods are also much higher in fructose than in glucose. How can you tell which foods have unhealthy carbs? Easy: they come in a box.

Of the 60,000 foods available in American grocery stores, over 80 percent have added fructose and processed carbohydrates. Most foods in the center of the grocery store are some combination of processed wheat flour, high fructose corn syrup, hydrogenated oils, salt, and artificial flavors and colorings. If something has an ingredient list of more than three to five items, don't bother reading the list; just put it back on the shelf.

when should you eat carbs?

Along with how fast they get absorbed, you should know whether your carbs go to fat or muscle, and this is determined by what time of day they are eaten. The Adrenal Reset Diet provides most of the day's carbs in the afternoon and evening. This is because at night, the muscles are more sensitive to insulin and they take the carbs before the fat gets to do so. Eating them at night also helps the body relax and repair the cycles leading to good sleep and fewer aches and pains.

protein and fat:
the remaining musketeers

As important as it is to get the carbs right, they can't do their magic unless they have the right amounts and the right types of protein and fat along with them.

protein

The word *protein* is derived from a Greek word meaning "first" or "primary." If we get enough protein, yet not much carbohydrate or fat, our health might suffer but we will survive. On the other hand, even with enough carbohydrate and fat, a lack of protein can be fatal. Diets that are extremely low in protein damage the intestines so badly that nothing can be absorbed.

Since few in the modern world lack protein badly enough to cause a fatal deficiency, many diet experts have argued that only the smallest amounts of protein are necessary. Yes, it takes very little protein to prevent a critical deficiency, but even with enough to prevent this, a diet can be so low in protein to cause the muscles, bones, and organs to slowly be used as additional sources of protein. In fact, this can even happen on a diet that is so high in calories that weight gain is occurring.[10]

which foods have protein?

High-quality protein foods include chicken, turkey, fish, shellfish, lean beef, buffalo, game meat, pork, and animal- or vegetable-based protein powder. Other foods that include protein are grains, beans, legumes, nuts, seeds, cheese, and milk. These latter foods do have protein but only as a small percentage of their total calories.

These lower-quality protein foods can prevent a protein deficiency but will not work as well as the higher-quality proteins for staying lean. This was shown in a fascinating study in which a group of twenty-five people were overfed 1,000 calories per day for eight weeks. They were divided into a vegetarian diet group getting 5 percent of their calories from protein; an average American diet group with 15 percent protein; and a high-protein diet group with 25 percent protein. Over the course of the study, each group gained weight, but the type of weight gained differed. The low-protein group lost 1.5 pounds of muscle, even though they gained fat. On the other hand, half of the weight gain in the high-protein group was in muscle.[11]

how much protein do you need?

To stay lean and keep a healthy metabolic rate, protein should make up roughly 25 to 30 percent of your calories. This means that one-fourth to one-third of your daily food volume should be from protein-rich foods.

where should you get your protein?

Among the high-protein foods, there are a few that should be given close consideration. Soy foods are best to be avoided as a regular protein source; they disrupt thyroid function, alter hormone metabolism, and promote weight gain.[12] Eggs and nonfat unsweetened Greek yogurt are great sources of protein, but because many people can't tolerant them, they are best avoided until you are well outside of survival mode.

With poultry, beef, and pork, the lower-fat choices are best. Of the many toxins we are exposed to, the worst ones that we cannot eliminate get stored in our fat. The animals we eat do the same thing. Although organic, free-range and hormone-free animals are preferable, even these types have more toxins in their fat than in their lean meat. Seafood is well documented to improve health, but considerations should be taken for purity and sustainability.

BEST CHOICES: Organic and free-range white- and dark-meat chicken, white- and dark-meat turkey, lean grass-fed beef; best seafoods are clams, oysters, scallops, shrimp, salmon (wild-caught), sardines, snapper.

fats—essential and nonessential

Most fats that the body uses can be made inside of us, as we need them; these are called *nonessential fats*. Other fats are essential for our health and we cannot make them. Like essential vitamins, we need to consume these on a regular basis to stay healthy. There are two types of essential fats: omega-3 and omega-6.

omega-3 fats

Omega-3 fats are critical for many aspects of good health, especially for the development and function of the brain and the control of inflammation. These fats include one vegetable omega-3 called *alpha linolenic acid* (ALA) and two animal omega-3 fats, called EPA and DHA. Due to genetic variation in an enzyme called *delta 5 desaturase*, about half of us can make vegetable omega-3 into EPA. However, omnivores like humans cannot make vegetable EPA into DHA. Because of this, animal omega-3 sources are best. As a backup for strict vegetarians, there are supplements that contain both EPA and DHA from algae.

BEST CHOICES: Good types of seafood mentioned under the protein "Best Choices" section, as well as vegetable omega-3s like flax and hemp.

omega-6 fats

Omega-6 fats are also called *linolenic acid*. They are essential for repairing the skin and making essential building blocks in the body, like the nerve cells. Our requirements for omega-6 fats are small, and we can easily get enough in our diets. Omega-6 fats are found in all nuts, seeds, and vegetable oils. Data have also suggested that, along with omega-3 and omega-6 being essential, they function best when they are found in certain ratios in the body.

Nuts and seeds can provide all of the needed omega-6 fats when you consume ¼ to ½ cup daily.

BEST CHOICES: Almonds, Brazil nuts, cashews, macadamia nuts, pistachios, avocados, pumpkin seeds, sunflower seeds, walnuts.

omega-9 fats

Omega-9 fats are not essential, although the foods that contain them may be high in fiber or have good chemicals like phenols. Omega-9 fats are also called *monounsaturated fats,* and they are found in olives, olive oil, almonds, avocados, macadamias, and pistachios. Once you have met your need for the essential fats, omega-9 foods are good sources for any remaining fat calories.

BEST CHOICES: Olives, olive oil, avocados.

saturated fats

For years, saturated fats were held out to be the villains causing heart disease and cancer. Many authors and researchers currently and in the recent past have pointed out the shortcomings of these arguments, however. Now, some nutritionists and doctors wonder if saturated fats are not only harmless but may be healthy.

Saturated fat is also called *palmitic acid.* All mammals, including humans, have the chemical ability to form palmitic acid from a variety of available building blocks. When we need it, we make it.

One of the strongest rules of nutrition is that we are healthiest when we have enough essential nutrients, but not too many unnecessary calories. Since saturated fats are not essential, pure sources like margarine, butter, sour cream, and cream add little to the diet beyond extra calories. These foods do not contain essential nutrients like protein, fiber, or vitamins, and so it is best to limit them. However, when saturated fats are in animal proteins, like dark-meat poultry or lean grass-fed beef, they are often accompanied by quality protein and many essential micronutrients.

BEST CHOICES: Dark-meat chicken, dark-meat turkey, grass-fed beef.

how much fat do you need?

Although our need for essential fats can be met with small quantities, if we eat too little fat we often end up eating too many carbs. For this reason, fats should make up between 20 and 35 percent of our calories. Fats are much more concentrated than protein or carbohydrates, so to get a third of your calories from fat requires much less than a third of your total food volume.

Many prepared foods already have enough, or even too much, added fat. When eating unprocessed foods that do not naturally contain fat, such as beans, whole grains, vegetables, lean proteins, and fruits, it is good to include some source of healthy fat. Each meal should have 1 to 2 tablespoons of nuts or nut butters, or 1 to 2 teaspoons of oil, or about one-fourth of a medium avocado.

but does it really work? results from the ARD study

After years of seeing this program work for individuals, I launched a formal study to determine how well it would work in a group. The intent was to show two things: that the diet leads to loss of visceral fat, and that it resets adrenal function.

My patients have always been like extended family to me, so when I asked for help with this, they turned out in a big way. For one month, a group of fifty-eight people followed the exact same Adrenal Reset Diet as you find in this book. In the study, there was one important difference, though. I wanted to show that the diet alone could flip the fat switch, as measured by daily cortisol rhythms. Because of this, I asked the participants not to change anything else about their lives besides their diet. They were asked not to take any herbal adaptogens or other supplements; not to increase their exercise habits; not to do relaxation techniques; and not to change their sleep habits.

Any of these additional steps would have made the results better and easier to maintain, but I wanted to see what we could accomplish with just *one* change. After the first month, I broadened the scope to include these other aspects of good health, but in that first month all the good changes came solely from the diet.

By the end of the study, forty-two participants had completed all of the weigh-ins and the pre- and post-testing. Their average age was 44, and 83 percent were female. Over the course of the month, their results were nothing short of remarkable. The greatest amount of weight lost was 18.2 pounds, while the average was just over 9 pounds. Only two participants did not lose weight, but even they saw a reduction in the percentage of body fat. Changes in waist measurements were also dramatic. Over half of the participants (22) lost over 2 inches around their waist. Several lost over 4 inches!

Changes in adrenal function from the diet were also clear. By measuring daily cortisol rhythms, we compared how close their adrenal function was to ideal, both before and after the study. Because when the adrenal glands do not work right the scores are just as apt to be too high as too low, we instead measured how much the scores differed from healthy levels.

The study showed that at all times of day the diet moved cortisol levels closer to their ideal amounts. *The average participant saw a correction of his or her whole day's cortisol metabolism by over 50 percent with diet.* (Isolated studies have shown that dietary changes influence cortisol, but I have not been able to find evidence of another diet being used to successfully restore the delicate circadian rhythm that governs our health.) The results of the study are shown in Table 3.2.

What does better cortisol metabolism mean? It means less belly fat, better energy, less anxiety, better depth of sleep, a healthier immune system, and a longer life. If you are in survival mode, carbohydrate cycling can start to move you out of it in as little as twenty-four hours. After thirty days of strategic carbohydrate cycling, your new healthy cortisol rhythm starts to become automatic and is even easier to maintain because it is your body's inherent rhythm. This rhythm allows for abundant energy and natural, easy weight loss.

TABLE 3.2. 30-DAY RESULTS OF ARD STUDY

BODY CHANGES	WEIGHT	BMI	FAT %	WAIST
Starting Average	182.3	29.4	35.42%	37.7
Ending Average	173.3	28.0	33.41%	35.6
Total Changes	-9.20	-1.46	-2%	-2.19
Percentage Change	-5.05%	-4.95%	-5.80%	-5.81%

ADRENAL CHANGES	TIME OF MEASUREMENT			
	7-9 AM	NOON-1 PM	5-6 PM	11 PM-MID
*Ideal Cortisol (nMol/L)	22.00	13.00	6.00	1
Average Variation Pre (nMol/L)	7.69	7.05	4.90	4.93
Average Variation Pos (nMol/L)	3.79	4.19	2.62	2.57
Average Changes (nMol/L)	3.90	2.86	2.29	2.36
Percentage Change	50.8%	40.5%	46.6%	47.8%

Total Variation Pre - 4 Scores Combined	24.57
Total Variation Post - 4 Scores Combined	13.17
Reduction in Cortisol Variation	53.59%

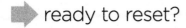 ready to reset?

The Adrenal Reset Diet is clinically proven and supported by science. In the next chapter, you will learn how easy it is and (as you've already seen) how it includes lots of foods you already love.

the adrenal
reset diet

THESE SIMPLE STEPS CAN GET THE BALL ROLLING AS YOU READ the rest of this book and learn about the rest of the program so that it becomes your own.

ARD meals

The Adrenal Reset Diet (ARD) does not require calorie counting. Instead, it has targeted portions for proteins, fats, and carbs. Throughout the day each meal has the same amounts of healthy proteins and fats. The only difference from one meal to the next is the number of servings of carbs: they increase throughout the day.

breakfast

Breakfast does not avoid carbs all together, but it has one small serving that is especially high in fiber. This morning serving of fiber is important for your adrenal reset. The best strategies for breakfast are either doing protein shakes or eating the same types of food you would eat at your other meals. Chicken, broccoli, and beans may sound like an unusual breakfast, but they can give you an unusually high metabolism! The idea of breakfast as a multi-carb event with cereal, juice, fruit, milk, and pastries just does not work.

lunch

Many people are busy, and lunch is often given little forethought. My favorite trick for lunch involves planning it the day before. When I'm making dinner, I make extra and pack some for lunch, with a palm-size serving of healthy starch. Some of your better options when eating out include soup with beans, a gluten-free turkey wrap, a salad with some kidney or garbanzo beans, or a stir-fry with ½ cup brown rice—nothing fried, and no sugary sauces.

dinner

Most people have the easiest time getting dinner right. Typical dinners already consist of a protein, a side dish of healthy carbs, and some vegetables. So the ARD dinner usually just involves choosing the healthiest versions of these foods and the best amounts. Eating more food by adding a little more healthy starch than you may normally have is a change that few have difficulty adopting.

snacks

These are optional. If you are in the habit of snacking and you prefer to continue doing so, think of snacks as a great time to eat a few extra servings of veggies. This can be as easy as having a bag of baby carrots and celery on hand. Another great option for snacks is juicing. Nutritionists universally agree that you can improve your health by eating more fresh vegetables, and juicing can help you get more veggies and also give you some tasty options for beverages if you are bored of water. The recipe chapter has some great juice blends for each of the adrenal levels as well as for specific health goals.

Until the most recent decades, people rarely snacked as they do now. We have been led to believe that something terrible will happen to us if we do not eat every few hours. But when you are thriving and healthy, it will not worry you to go several hours between meals and to eat fewer times per day. As you get there, a handful of baby carrots can tide you over. If you are worried about gaining weight from eating less, see "How Many Times Per Day Should I Eat?" on page 244.

 ## carb cycling for weight loss

We gain weight because modern life disrupts our adrenal rhythms and puts us in survival mode. But our food choices can act as a tool to reset this rhythm. The Adrenal Reset Diet is the first plan to strategically use the carb/cortisol response to systematically cycle carbohydrates for weight loss.

protein for breakfast

Whenever people tell me they struggle with weight gain, the very first question I ask is what they eat for breakfast. There may be no single meal that is more important. Unfortunately, many people skip breakfast all together, or they have a carb-a-thon of pancakes, waffles, juices, syrup, muffins, and pastries. Food like this creates a spike in blood sugar, forcing the morning cortisol to plummet. This sets a person up for a day of being edgy, out of focus, and unable to burn fat. The other problem with breakfast foods is that the few that are not processed carbs often have toxic proteins, like dairy and eggs. Eating the traditional carbo-laden breakfast means that for the rest of the day you will feel less energized, you will store fat more easily, and you will have poorer quality sleep at night.

ARD breakfasts focus on high-quality protein, alkalizing vegetables, high amounts of fiber, and moderate amounts of healthy fats. You will notice that there are some carbs, like lentils, white beans, pinto beans, and green peas, that have been included. These are intentionally used owing to their high amounts of naturally occurring resistant fiber (their F:F ratio). Gluten-free, old-fashioned rolled oats and bananas are also included in some recipes. Both are used raw, and the bananas are better when they are a little bit unripe, with some green on their peels. These carbs metabolize so slowly you can eat them for breakfast and not absorb the carbs until afternoon!

A breakfast and lunch that are higher in protein can support the healthy morning spike of cortisol. This gives you energy for both your muscles and your brain. It also allows you to burn fat for fuel and keep your blood sugar levels stable throughout the day.[1]

balanced lunch

Later in the day, it is a different story. Ideally, your cortisol will start lowering after lunch as your insulin starts to rise. Lunch is a good time to have ½ cup of healthy carbs to initiate the cortisol reduction, so you can eventually get to needed nighttime levels. Energy production and mental focus will be critical for several more hours, so the best lunch contains balanced amounts of protein, starch, and fat.

A lunch with less than ½ cup carbohydrate would keep up the morning energy peak but would also require cortisol to stay high to keep the blood sugar levels up. On the other hand, if lunch has too many carbohydrates your brain goes into sleep mode, which is not helpful for your day.

healthy carbs at night

By dinnertime, your insulin response is at its peak. If you do not have some carbohydrates, cortisol will raise your blood sugar, which will prevent your getting a good night's sleep.[2] This can also cause a blood sugar crash, which leads to sugar cravings.

By testing glucose levels minute by minute throughout the night in hundreds of people, I have observed that unstable blood sugar levels occur exactly when people are struggling to fall asleep or are spontaneously waking up at night. Carb cycling helps keep the cortisol levels where they should be during the day but is critical to keeping them low enough at night to allow for deep sleep.[3]

magic portions to heal your proportions

Here are the best sources for protein, fat, and carbs, as well as what a good serving size is for each. Please note that these amounts do not necessarily correspond with the serving sizes on food labels.

protein

When choosing protein-rich foods, focus on those that are least processed, that are organic, and that are lowest in salt. The largest source of pesticide residues in the average diet comes from animal fat. For this reason, animal products that have fat should be given the highest priority in your budget choices for organic foods.

Each serving of protein should be the size of the palm of your hand, or 4 to 6 ounces.

Beef, lean grass-fed

Beef, lean ground grass-fed

Black cod / sablefish

Canadian bacon, nitrate-free—3 pieces

Chicken breast

Cod

Crab meat

Ham, lean, nitrate-free

Lamb chop

Lamb loin

Lamb, rack

Lobster

Oysters

Pork chop, lean

Pork loin, lean

Protein powder, vegetable-based (1 serving)

Salmon, wild-caught Alaskan

Sardines

Shrimp

Turkey bacon, nitrate-free—3 pieces

Turkey breast

Turkey, deli meat, nitrate-free

Turkey, ground

Trout, rainbow

fats

The best sources of healthy fats are raw nuts and seeds. These are easy to keep in the pantry and regularly include in your meals. Nuts and seeds all have very specific nutrient profiles. For example, Brazil nuts are very high in selenium, almonds are very high in magnesium. So it is good to have several different types in the diet and to rotate among them regularly.

Almonds—¼ cup

Almond butter—2 tablespoons

Avocado—⅓ medium

Brazil nuts*—¼ cup

Chia seeds—2 tablespoons or ¾ ounce

Canola oil—1 tablespoon

Coconut, shredded unsweetened—2 tablespoons

Coconut oil—1 tablespoon

Flax seeds—2 tablespoons

Guacamole—3 tablespoons

Hemp seeds—2 tablespoons

Macadamia nuts—¼ cup

Macadamia oil—1 tablespoon

Olive oil—1 tablespoon

Olives—½ cup

Pistachios, unsalted and shelled—¼ cup

Pumpkin seeds— 2 tablespoons

Sesame oil, toasted— 1 tablespoon

Sunflower seeds— 2 tablespoons

Walnuts—¼ cup

Vegan-type mayonnaise— 2 tablespoons

carbohydrates

Carbs are best when they come from vegetables, fruits, intact whole grains, and beans. Some good staples to keep on hand are frozen fruit and veggies, low-sodium canned beans, and pre-cooked

* Limit to once weekly to prevent selenium overdose.

brown rice and quinoa. These are all helpful to have ready-to-go for last-minute meals.

Acorn squash—¼ cup cooked

Adzuki beans—¼ cup cooked

Barley—¼ cup cooked

Beets—¼ cup cooked

Black beans—¼ cup cooked

Blackberries—¼ cup

Blueberries—¼ cup

Brown rice—¼ cup cooked

Butternut squash—
¼ cup cooked

Cannellini beans—
¼ cup cooked

Corn kernels—¼ cup cooked

Garbanzo beans
(chickpeas)—¼ cup cooked

Grapefruit—¼ medium

Great northern beans—
¼ cup cooked

Hummus—2 tablespoons

Kidney beans—¼ cup cooked

Kabocha squash—
¼ cup cooked

Lentils—¼ cup cooked

Navy beans—¼ cup cooked

Parsnips—¼ cup boiled

Peas—¼ cup cooked

Peach—½ medium

Pinto beans—¼ cup cooked

Potato—¼ cup boiled

Quinoa—¼ cup cooked

Raspberries—¼ cup

Gluten-free old-fashioned
rolled oats—¼ cup raw

Strawberries—¼ cup

Sweet potato—
¼ cup cooked

Turnips—¼ cup cooked

IF YOU ARE TRYING FOR FASTER WEIGHT LOSS, LIMIT THE FOLLOW-
ING CARBS TO A FEW TIMES PER WEEK OR LESS:

Apple—½ medium

Banana—½ medium

Cantaloupe melon—
½ cup cubed

Honeydew melon—
½ cup cubed

Pear—½ medium

Plums—1 medium

Kiwi—½

Mango—¼ cup cubed

Orange—½ medium

Pasta, gluten-free—
¼ cup cooked

Pineapple—¼ cup cubed

Plantain—¼ cup cooked

Nectarine—½ medium

Watermelon—½ cup cubed

UNLIMITED FOODS: HAVE AS MUCH AS YOU WANT,
WHENEVER YOU WANT

Alfalfa sprouts

Artichokes, artichoke
hearts

Asparagus

Bamboo shoots

Bean sprouts

Bok choy, baby bok choy

Broccoli

Brussels sprouts

Cabbage

Carrots

Cauliflower

Celery

Celery root

Collard greens

Cucumbers

Daikon

Eggplant

Fennel

Garlic

Ginger

Green beans

Green onions, scallions

Jicama

Kale

Kohlrabi

Leeks

Lemon juice

Lettuce greens: green leaf,
red leaf, butter, romaine,
radicchio

Lime juice

Mushrooms

Okra

Onions

Peppers, green and red

Radishes

Rutabaga

Salad greens: chicory, endive, escarole, arugula, watercress

Snow peas

Spinach

Sugar snap pea pods

Summer squash: crookneck, zucchini

Sunflower sprouts

Swiss chard

Tomatoes

Tomatillos

Turnip greens

Water chestnuts

Winter squash: spaghetti, pumpkin

weight loss in the palm of your hand . . .

When you are on the go, here is a trick to make eyeballing your portion sizes easier. Think about each meal's protein serving (like fish or poultry) as the same size as the palm of your hand. For each meal, have as much healthy fat (like nuts or avocados) as would be the size of a golf ball. For carbs, eat a golf ball-size serving for breakfast, two golf ball-size servings for lunch, and three golf ball-size servings for dinner.

MASTER YOUR SERVINGS

	Breakfast	Lunch	Dinner
Protein	Palm of your hand		
Fat	Golf ball		
Carbs	1 golf ball	2 golf balls	3 golf balls

eating is as easy as 1–2–3

Remember the Jackson Five's song about falling in love being as easy as "one-two-three"? Now that you know your building blocks, attaining weight loss is just as easy. Each meal is one serving each of fat and protein. Carbs are *1* serving for breakfast, *2* for lunch, and *3* for dinner. Easy as *1–2–3*! Here's the ARD in menu form:

MEALS	SERVINGS
Breakfast	1 serving protein 1 serving fat 1 servings carbs—legumes, resistant starch, or berries [Foods from unlimited list in any quantity]
Lunch	1 serving protein 1 serving fat 2 servings carbs [Foods from unlimited list in any quantity]
Dinner	1 serving protein 1 serving fat 3 servings carbs [Foods from unlimited list in any quantity]
Mid-morning and mid-afternoon snacks	[Foods from unlimited list in any quantity]

a quickstart menu

The ARD can be as simple or as gourmet as you wish. For the ultimate in simplicity, think of it as the 3 Ss: *Shake*, *Salad*, and *Stir-fry*. Here are some basic ideas to get you started:

breakfast: shake

Some of the shake ingredients are nontraditional but strategic for the reset, and they have no negative taste impact.

basic shake

Serves 2

> 2 servings sugar-free, animal- or vegetable-based protein powder
>
> ¼ cup frozen berries
>
> 1 cup unsweetened flax milk
>
> 2 tablespoons flax seeds
>
> 1 small handful frozen spinach
>
> ¼ cup cooked navy beans

Blend all the ingredients in a high-powered blender with ½ cup each ice cubes and water.

lunch: salad

Remember that many vegetables are on the unlimited list, so eat up!

basic salad

½ cup cooked black beans

1 palm-size serving canned salmon

Several handfuls of romaine, red leaf, or green leaf lettuce

1 large handful cherry tomatoes

1 tablespoon olive oil

½ teaspoon red wine vinegar

½ teaspoon Spike brand seasoning blend (available in most
   supermarkets)

Rinse the beans, and fork the salmon; place in a large bowl. Add the remaining ingredients and mix well. Keep chilled until ready to serve.

dinner: stir-fry

Who has time to make dinner? You do, when it's as easy as this.

basic stir-fry

Both rice and chicken breast can be purchased precooked or can be cooked in advance.

2 teaspoons toasted sesame oil
1 garlic clove, minced
½ cup diced onion
1 large handful broccoli florets
1 small handful sliced button mushrooms
1 teaspoon grated fresh ginger
¾ cup cooked brown rice
1 palm-size serving cooked chicken breast
1 teaspoon soy sauce

Heat half the oil in a saucepan or wok. Cook the garlic and onion for about 1 minute. Add the vegetables and ginger, and cook until lightly soft, about 5 minutes. Add the rice, chicken, soy sauce, and remaining 1 teaspoon sesame oil and stir, heating until all ingredients are warm.

➡ have it your way

If you tire of the basic recipe combinations, or just don't like one of the ingredients in them, here are some really easy ways to add variety without adding much complexity.

breakfast shake substitutions

- Instead of flax milk, use unsweetened coconut milk or almond milk.

- Use chia, hemp, salvia, or pumpkin seeds instead of flax seeds.

- Substitute kale, collards, or other greens for the spinach.

salad substitutions

- You can use any other greens in place of the lettuce.

- Try another type of bean; garbanzo (chickpeas) and navy beans are great options.

- Chicken, shrimp, tempeh, or other protein-rich foods can be used in place of the salmon.

- Use any other vinegar, with the exception of flavored or balsamic vinegar. If you are not sure if a vinegar is flavored, just check the label; if total carbs are over 1 gram per serving, it is likely flavored.

- Other oils can be used in place of olive oil, such as macadamia or rice bran oil.

- Other seasoning blends can replace Spike, such as herbes de Provence, Italian seasoning mix, lemon pepper, or Mrs. Dash seasoning blend.

stir-fry substitutions

- Any other nonstarchy vegetables can be used, in unlimited amounts.

- Try lean beef, pork, or tempeh instead of chicken.

- Other oils can replace the toasted sesame oil. Macadamia oil works well in stir-fries.

- Other seasonings can be substituted for the soy sauce. Although soy itself is avoided, tamari soy sauce is wheat-free, fermented, and fine for use in typical quantities. Ume plum vinegar is a great substitute.

 # where are you today?

Now that you know how foods can reset your adrenals and restart your fat switch, learn how some simple lifestyle tricks can help your fat loss go even faster and last over the long term.

Remember that the three problems associated with obesity are processed food, pollutants, and life's pressures. The Adrenal Reset Diet eliminates the effects of processed foods and much of the effects of pollutants. Along with this, restoring your circadian rhythm and gaining clearer thinking will help you thrive—in no time. These additional steps really shine if they are matched to your current needs. So, are you Stressed, Wired and Tired, Crashed, or already Thriving? Let's find out by taking the quiz in the next chapter.

learn your level

and go from surviving to thriving

AS MENTIONED IN EARLIER CHAPTERS, THE MAIN THREE PROB-lems underlying the obesity crisis are processed food, a polluted world, and the pressures of daily life. These three elements of modern living tend to flip the AFS from thriving to survival mode.

The Adrenal Reset Diet can reset the switch and make weight loss happen naturally. If you have a lot of ongoing adrenal stress, though, that can hamper success, especially for the long term. The following Adrenal Level Quiz will help you assess what level of adrenal function you have and what specific ways you can improve that function. Doing so will help your weight loss go faster, take less effort, and last longer. These steps will also help you sleep better, have more energy, and enjoy life more—you'll thrive even during times the inevitable stressors come your way.

Recognizing your adrenal level helps tremendously, as each level responds best to a different strategy. In essence, what works well for one will not work as well for another. The idea that there are these four levels dates back to the earliest concepts of stress, as it was first identified by a researcher named Hans Selye. He discovered that, as survival mode worsens, it moves through a series of distinct and predictable levels. As the stress is lowered and health returns, the same levels show up in reverse order. The following is an overview of these levels of stress.

the stressed level

Selye called the first level the *alarm*. This is like the reaction to a loud noise or a fearful scene. During alarm the heart speeds up, more blood moves to the muscles, and the body gets ready to run or fight. The adrenal glands are making extra cortisol to allow the person to respond to this danger. The state can also be triggered by social anxiety, public speaking, worry over the kids, feeling over-whelmed and overly busy, or performance-related events, such as presenting a project to the boss or taking a test.

Many people today find themselves spending time in the state of alarm on a daily basis. Since this condition shares many symptoms with what we commonly think of as "stressed" today, I've renamed the level "Stressed" to reflect that more recognizable state. In Chapter 6 you will learn that this state is helped by foods and simple tricks, which can improve your sense of relaxation throughout the day.

 the wired and tired level

If the event triggering the alarm is lasting, like hunger or extreme cold, the body will do its best to adjust to it. Selye called this *resistance*. At this level, the body is putting so much energy into resisting that it is less able to maintain health. The adrenal glands are making extra cortisol, and their daily rhythm has been disrupted. Although resistance can have many ever-changing symptoms, the core feeling is urgency paired with a sense of weakness. I find that the phrase "Wired and Tired" captures this well. Those at this level need foods and habits that rebuild daytime energy and establish nighttime relaxation. These are covered in Chapter 7.

 the crashed level

If the stress causing resistance does not let up, health clearly be-comes compromised. Selye called this stage *exhaustion*. At this point, symptoms get worse and they persist. The adrenal glands have made so many extra hormones for so long that now they cannot make enough to meet the body's daily needs. What also happens is that diseases of adaptation, like high blood sugar, high blood pressure, allergies, digestive problems, and depression, can get a foothold. Exhaustion is typified by a deep feeling of weakness and collapse. Since it represents a point at which one is forced to slow down, I call this level "Crashed." If you are crashed, you need gentle support to enhance the energy production throughout the day, as discussed in Chapter 8.

Table 5.1 shows these three levels as contrasted with the fourth level, Thriving.

TABLE 5.1. ADRENAL LEVELS—AN OVERVIEW

	THRIVING	SURVIVING		
		STRESSED	WIRED	CRASHED
How you feel	Enthusiastic	Edgy	Overwhelmed	Exhausted
How other people seem to you	Engaging	Too slow	Incompetent	Demanding
Your sleep is	Deep and restful	Hard to fall asleep	Hard to stay asleep	Unrefreshing
Your mental function is	Sharp and focused	Fast and scattered	Erratic	Unable to generate ideas
Best type of exercise is	Any, have fun	Strength training	Cardio	Yoga

the adrenal level quiz

Where are you today along this continuum? This easy quiz will help you find out. Take it now and repeat it monthly to track your journey back to thriving. If you are not happy with your results, know that the tips in the chapter for your current level can guide you in the right direction. With the Adrenal Reset Diet and these tricks designed for your level, you truly can heal and thrive!

Directions: For each symptom, rate a response from 0 to 3, based on how often you experience it.

0 = Never
1 = Weekly
2 = Daily
3 = Several times per day

SECTION 1

____ Anxiety
____ Depression
____ Frequent urination
____ Fidgety
____ Hard to concentrate
____ Headaches
____ Irritability
____ Jaw pain or teeth grinding
____ Lack of joy or enthusiasm
____ Diminished memory
____ Picking at skin or fingernails
____ Poor sleep
____ Sighing frequently
      Section 1 total = _____

SECTION 2

____ Allergies worsening

____ Blurred vision

____ Blood pressure too low or too high

____ Fatigue throughout the day

____ Facial swelling

____ Heart rate rapid even when resting

____ Intolerance to cold weather

____ Mid-body weight gain

____ Muscle cramps

____ Muscular weakness

____ Neck stiffness

____ Sensitivity to bright lights

____ Shaking hands

Section 2 total = _____

SECTION 3

____ Caffeine *needed* each morning

____ Frequent constipation

____ Cravings for heavy or fatty foods

____ Frequent dehydration

____ Fatigue in the afternoon

____ Gas and bloating

____ Regular heartburn

____ Irregular stools

____ Irritability when meals are delayed

____ Joint pain

____ Nausea

____ Salt cravings

____ Sugar cravings

Section 3 total = _____

Total Stress Load (Section 1+2+3) = _____

QUIZ RESULTS

0–15 = Thriving
16–30 = Stressed
31–45 = Wired and Tired
46+ = Crashed

 what does your score mean?

If your category is Stressed, your body is still vital but a steady survival mode may be affecting your weight. The steps in Chapter 6 will allow you to lose weight more easily, feel more relaxed, and be less apt to regain weight when life gets hectic.

If your category is Wired and Tired, stress is now likely causing some clear changes in your energy and mood. Chapter 7 will help your sleep become a time in which you can repair your body and start breaking down fat stores. Your daytime energy levels will become more steady and predictable.

If your category is Crashed, your health may be starting to suffer. Substantial rest and recovery are needed. Chapter 8 will greatly increase your energy and your ability to exercise. You will also notice better mental clarity and a newfound ability to stick with the plans that you know can help.

do you need a lab test?

It is helpful for you and your doctor to be aware of your corti-sol levels, and a number of lab tests are available to evaluate cortisol function. Be aware, though, that their findings may not match your quiz results. The shortcoming of current tests is that they all reflect circulating cortisol made from the adrenals, not whole-body cortisol that includes that made by the fat, liver, and brain. Whole-body cortisol levels can be measured in research studies, but they cannot be measured by routine medical labs.

Even so, salivary cortisol tests can be a good way to look at circadian rhythms and chart your progress as your health im-proves. For more information about adrenal testing, visit www .adrenalresetdiet.com/resources.

 easy steps for every stress level

Here are a few simple steps that can be helpful to anyone, regardless of current stress level.

step 1. make sure your thyroid is happy

If your thyroid levels are not at their best, your body may be storing hundreds of extra calories each day. Although thyroid disease can affect anyone, some are especially at risk. Those most at risk for thy-roid disease include:

- Females

- People over 40

- Those with a family history of thyroid disease

- Women with a past use of oral contraceptives

- Those with a history of unsuccessful dieting

If you are already on thyroid treatment, thyroid disease can still be a factor making any weight loss harder. Based on a large national survey conducted by thyroid patient advocate Mary Shomon in 2001, the majority of people on treatment are not on the best dose of the best medicine for their weight.

How can you know if thyroid function may be a factor in your weight gain? There is a detailed quiz with simple action steps at www.adrenalresetdiet.com/resources.

step 2. bone up on vitamin D3 and magnesium

VITAMIN D

Vitamin D is important for your bones and immune system. It turns out that it is also critical for weight loss and good blood sugar control. The more stable your blood sugar is, the healthier your adrenal glands are. A large study showed that adult women with vitamin D levels below 30 ng/ml were at higher risk for weight gain and diabetes.[1]

In theory, we should get enough vitamin D from the sun. Our skin has cells that work along with naturally occurring oils to form vitamin D when we are in the sun. Yet because we are often indoors, wear clothes and sunscreen, and frequently wash off our natural oils, most people do not get enough vitamin D.

How much vitamin D should you take in supplements and of what type? Not everyone needs the same dose, so it's best to talk with your physician to decide what's right for you. Vitamin D is best absorbed when taken with a meal that contains some healthy fats, and vitamin D3 is the preferred form because of its better absorption. Most adults can safely start with 2,000 IU daily. Ideally, though, you should have your blood levels of vitamin D tested every three months until they fall between 50 and 80 ng/ml. Once the levels are stable, it is good to test once per year.

Individual needs vary, so a healthy level may take a dose of anywhere between 2,000 and 10,000 IU. It is important also to supplement with 100 percent of the recommended daily allowance (RDA) of vitamins K, E, and A when taking vitamin D, as they all work together. Adults can safely take 1,000 IU per day of vitamin D without testing, but this may not be enough for you. If you are pregnant, elderly, have kidney disease, or are on certain medications, your needs may vary. Speak with your doctor to find your perfect dose.

MAGNESIUM

Your adrenal glands need magnesium to work right.[2] As important as this is, 68 percent of Americans do not get enough magnesium.[3] Common problems like stress, obesity, and pre-diabetes make people even more apt to be low in magnesium.[4] When supplementing with magnesium, it seems that most types, like magnesium oxide or magnesium citrate, can work fine. A good dose is between 250 and 600 mg daily, taken with food. Note: although everyone gets loose stools if they take too much magnesium, some people have this happen even with normal doses.

SELECTING SUPPLEMENTS

Since getting the right nutrients is critical for both weight loss and adrenal health, it is important to avoid any barriers to effectiveness. The biggest obstacles can be how well the nutrients are absorbed, how pure they are, how convenient they are to take, and whether or not they have synthetic additives and fillers.

Poor-quality supplements may not be absorbed and may simply produce expensive urine or stools. Better supplements are manufactured to meet guidelines set by the U.S. Food and Drug Administration (FDA), the Natural Products Association (NPA), the National Sanitary Foundation (NSF), and the Australian Therapeutic Goods Administration (TGA). These guidelines ensure that what you take is free of harmful additives and that the ingredients end up in your bloodstream.

For detailed reviews and information on currently used adrenal supplements, visit www.adrenalresetdiet.com/resources.

step 3. detox daily: the three easiest ways to clear pollutants

Your body eliminates chemicals in a two-stage process. In the first stage, they are "activated" so they are ready to move. In the second stage, they are "conjugated." Think of the latter as being packed in a box for safe shipping. The big dilemma with detoxification attempts is that certain toxins, like plastics and solvents, alter the attempts. Many of them speed up the first stage and slow down the second stage. When this happens, it makes them even more dangerous, and we don't eliminate them.

The following are ways to detoxify.

BROCCOLI SPROUTS

One of the few things that can help with detoxification is a compound from vegetables called *sulfurophane*. This substance is found in broccoli, cauliflower, Brussels sprouts, and cabbage. And along with helping with weight loss and detoxification, sulfurophane has been shown to lower the risk of developing many cancers. Broccoli is great, but if you really want easy weight loss, upgrade to broccoli sprouts. They have up to fifty times as much sulfurophane, and they are delicious. They can be easily added to salads or blended into smoothies. Adding one package of broccoli sprouts to your intake per week can clean the toxins out of your fat so you can shed that fat more easily.

RICE BRAN

A problem with chemical pollutants is that they just don't know when the party is over. We send them to our colon to leave the body but many get reabsorbed before leaving in the stool and sneak right back in. Rice bran fiber (RBF) acts like a bouncer at the door to make sure they stay gone for good.

How do you get enough RBF? Eating brown rice is great, but the amounts used in most studies to prove its worth are a little higher, typically 1/2 to 1 tablespoon. Thankfully, pure RBF can be found in most health food markets. A single tablespoon per day can multiply your body's elimination of toxins from plastics by 6.6 times.[5] The easiest way to take RBF is to add it to your morning shake. It has no major impact on taste or texture.

GROUND FLAX SEEDS

You may have heard that bacteria have been engineered to clean up oil spills. The same thing occurs in our bodies. The bacteria in the colon perform a critical part of detoxification. When the bacteria

> ## simple detox strategy:
>
> Broccoli sprouts—1 package per week
> Rice bran—1 tablespoon per day
> Ground flax seeds—1 tablespoon per day

are healthy, they break down the chemicals that we are trying to get rid of, especially chemicals that hurt our hormone balance. Flax seeds contain lignans that make those bacteria even better at this task. Ground flax seeds are the type that works best for this. Flax oil and whole flax seeds are fine for other things, but not a great source of lignans. Usually 1 to 2 tablespoons per day of ground flax seeds can improve your elimination of toxins such as pesticides.

step 4. create your perfect day

Melanie has been a dear friend and a patient for more than fifteen years. She is a hard-driving professional who quickly moved up the ranks in a Fortune 500 company. Her life is so busy that in the past she did not keep up with her health care. Her joke was that she came in to see me every twenty-four months, whether she needed it or not. It was a joke because she was always in distress and past due for a checkup. On one visit, she came with two big pieces of news: she had gained 32 pounds and she was now a vice president. Aware that her parents had both died from diabetes, she made a morbid joke about being on the fast track to becoming a rich dead lady.

I asked her to take a few minutes and describe her typical day to me. She explained that she slept four to five hours "on a good night" during her workweek, and tried to catch up on the weekends. She rarely ate breakfast and her days started two or three time zones earlier, since she lived on the West Coast but worked with an East Coast team. Each night she responded to emails and watched financial news until midnight or later.

Knowing that Melanie's capacity for change was limited by her responsibilities, I wanted to find the smallest steps that would give her the most benefit. I asked her for just three changes in the next month: First, she was to outsource the email and financial research. Second, she was to eat breakfast each morning with at least 25 grams of protein. And the third was that each night she would to turn off everything but a reading light by 9 PM. By the end of the month, Melanie was down 9 pounds without dieting or exercising. She was so excited she called to let me know.

Like Melanie, many people are pleasantly surprised that weight loss can be no harder than a few simple adjustments to daily habits. Good or bad, we all have daily habits. Do yours raise your total stress load or lower it? What are the easiest new habits you can start today that would make the most difference for you? What would your perfect day entail? Consider your responsibilities and your available time. Then look at the suggestions that follow for more ideas on crafting an adrenal-nourishing habit.

WAKE UP GENTLY

Your day's circadian rhythm gets started when you wake up. What happens then can completely control how the rest of the day plays out. Loud noises trigger a startle response that wakes you up certainly, but they also set off your internal alarm, which makes the day's stressors more intense.

If you cannot let yourself wake up naturally, there are alarm clocks that work like natural sunlight. They turn on fifteen to twenty minutes before you want to wake up and they gradually get brighter and brighter. Waking to bright light in this fashion has been shown to improve cortisol metabolism, which can make weight loss easier.[6]

Another gentle way to wake up is what I call the "reverse alarm." You use white noise during the night and shut it off when you want to wake up. Many white noise apps or generators have timers that can be set to turn off at a given time. Ideally, the white noise is low volume and constant. (Background noise that is loud and erratic is less helpful.)

ENJOY A CUP: RELAX WITH YOUR MORNING RITUALS

Waking up is more of a gradual transition than it may seem. Our brains take about an hour or so to deal reasonably well with the outside world—and for some this can take even longer. The time can be well spent in contemplation, in making plans, and in doing relaxation exercises. Even just a few quiet moments with a hot cup of herbal tea, tea, or coffee can set up the day in a good way. (And, for people with typical caffeine metabolism, coffee does not elevate cortisol in the morning.) Since TVs and computer screens speed the brain waves, they are not a good fit for early morning.[7] Give yourself at least an hour to get ready for the day's pace.

CALM YOUR COMMUTE

Surveys have shown that the morning commute may be the most stressful part of a person's day. Even if this is time you cannot change, you can still make it restorative. Do you travel 10 miles or less? You might be surprised how easy it is to bike to work some days. Bike a few days and use the driving days to bring fresh clothes and food in advance.

If a drive is inevitable, this can be golden time for personal growth and learning. There are so many great books and programs on audio now. Stress is reduced by healthy distractions and by receiving new ideas. Wouldn't it be great to learn a new language, deepen your knowledge of your mind and body, or learn to communicate better?

DISCONNECT AND RECONNECT

Each night our ancestors sought out companionship, substantial food, and warmth. Even today, evening is the best time to connect with loved ones and enjoy a hearty meal together. Although we often substitute "imagined interactions" via TV or "virtual interactions" via social media, real interactions are best.

step 5. sleep tight

Before we move onto the next chapter, it's important to discuss another daily habit that is crucial to your success: sleep.

is your sleep debt larger than the national debt?

How many hours of unbroken sleep have you averaged in the last thirty days? Take this number and multiply it by 30. Then, subtract that number from 240. The result is your current sleep debt. It turns out that repaying your sleep debt takes more than a single night. If your sleep debt is under 20 hours, sleep in for 9 hours total two nights in a row. If your debt is 20 to 40 hours, plan on 8 to 9 hours of sleep Monday to Friday, with naps of 2 to 3 hours each day on the weekend to get caught up. If your debt is over 40 hours, a "sleepcation" could change your life. This is where you check into a hotel for three nights, dim the room as much as possible, avoid stimulants, and let yourself sleep day and night.

A realtor I know once had a sleep debt of over 100 hours. Along with struggling with her weight, she complained that her career was falling apart because she could not remember any-thing and felt no motivation. The first month after her sleepca-tion, she dropped 12 pounds effortlessly and had the best sales quarter of her twenty-year career. It's not magic. Adequate sleep is critical for your health and performance.

What is more important for weight loss—diet or exercise? The real answer might be sleep. Sleep determines how much you eat, which foods you crave, and what your body does with the calories. To get into a bit of basic brain science, your ability to make good choices comes from your prefrontal cortex (PFC). You want to uti-lize that ability for making good choices.

As an example, think about the effects of alcohol, which acts on the PFC. Does it cause people to make better choices or worse choices? Sleep deprivation works just like alcohol. Should you have a bite of the cake to be polite, or should you have two pieces because it tastes so good? How you decide is strongly based on how well you have been sleeping.

Sleep also controls your insulin sensitivity. People who sleep less than normal, even for a few nights, have a 30 percent decrease in insulin response. This means they are getting 30 percent more fat and 30 percent less energy from the same food! The magic number that seems to clearly predict weight gain and poor health is roughly 7.5 hours. Many do well with more, but almost no one does well with less.

How much sleep is best for you? Think about how much you get after several days of being on vacation. (The first few days of a vacation, or weekend days, may not be a good gauge, since you may be catching up on lost sleep.)

JUST CHILL OUT

A factor that may be disrupting your circadian cycle is climate control. Our daily cycles prepare us for colder evenings, but they only work properly when we get cold at night. How do you chill out? You set your thermostat to the mid-60s at night and take a lukewarm shower before bed. Advanced therapies like ice bathing and whole-body cryotherapy can also help metabolism.[8]

GET CHARGED

If sleep does not come easy, one of the simplest steps to try, regardless of your level, is to use negative ions.

Have you ever been entranced by a campfire or notice the air after a rain? If so, you have experienced negative ions. These are charged particles in the air that are present in many natural settings. Negative ions have been well documented to improve sleep cycles, elevate mood, and lower appetite.[9, 10, 11]

To get the benefits of negative ions, expose yourself to as much fresh air as possible. Negative ions are more present in areas with more water and more vegetation. Spending time gardening can be particularly effective. Since moving water generates ions, relaxing in the shower can also give you a good dose of them. Negative ion generators are also readily available and inexpensive. Placed by your bedside, they can make the air seem like that of a fresh ocean breeze and may let you sleep better.

PEN, PAPER, AND PURPOSE

In the evening, our brains are trying to move the day's experiences into long-term memory, so it is natural to revisit the events and re-hash them. This is a good time for reflection and journaling. Dim the lights, get comfortable, and make some notes. Let your thoughts flow naturally, and write down any steps that require future action.

When you train yourself to do this each evening, your unresolved thoughts will stop intruding on your valuable sleep time. Reading something lighthearted or inspirational is also a great habit before bed. Remember how TVs and computers throw off the brain waves? Well, it appears that liquid ink readers, like the text-only versions of Kindle and Nook, do not cause this problem.

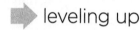 ## leveling up

Now that you know your adrenal level, and have some basic tips on maximizing sleep and your environment each day, you can dive into your chapter level for easy ways to supercharge your weight-loss success. In these chapters you will learn:

- How to best apply strategic carb cycling and the Adrenal Reset Diet to your stress level

- How to use level-specific ways to reset your circadian rhythm with proper detoxing, exercise, sleep, and herbal adaptogens

- How to gain mental clarity despite the pressures of everyday life

As you learn the tricks of the trade, here is a warning: do not identify too much with your level. After a little time following the ARD and practicing the habits for your level, you will find your Adrenal Level Quiz score getting higher; you will no longer be at the same level. This is great! As you move up, staying lean and healthy will become automatic.

How quickly your stress level changes depends on several factors, including your general health, the number and severity of life stressors you are experiencing, and your capacity for change. Typically, major improvements in metabolism and health can show up even in the first few days. Changes in your adrenal levels can happen from within a few weeks to a few months. But regardless of the time it takes, you'll move from your current stress level to that of thriving.

stressed

WHAT MOVES US FURTHER ALONG THE STRESS CONTINUUM IS HOW intense our stressors are, how long they last, and how many of them we deal with at once. Other big factors include our perceived control over events, our understanding of them, and how predictable they are.

You can move from Thriving to the Stressed level in a matter of days when prompted by events like minor financial pressures, changes at work, or conflicts with acquaintances. Apart from major catastrophes, the total number of stressors we face and how long they last are what matter most. Factors like processed foods and environmental pollutants can add to this total stress burden.

what happens when you're stressed

When you are stressed, you may have symptoms that indicate something is not right, although it is often not clear where they are coming from. Stress can cause symptoms such as:

- Racing heart

- Muscle twitches

- Headaches

- Fatigue

- Stomach pain or cramping

- Erratic bowel movements

- Sweating

- Muscle pain or tension

- Dizziness

allison's story: an insider's look at "stressed"

Allison "hated" her shape so much she said that if someone told her eating sawdust would fix it, she would do it. She had tried several diets and always had the same thing happen. She would lose a couple of pounds the first few weeks and then end up regaining, even though she was still on the program. Once she was able to unpack her frustrations about this, she shared with me how hectic her life had become.

When I asked her how her days went, she said they are all a big blur of stress. Each morning when the alarm goes off, she awakes feeling as if she did not sleep. Before getting out of bed, her mind rushes back to the same recurrent thoughts that kept her up the night before. Mostly, she worries about work and who will be let go of next; the work situation is only getting worse. Along with the layoffs, she is now doing the work three people used to do. Following in close second are her fears of needing new clothes if she gets any heavier. Adding to this, getting the kids fed and off to school is always chaotic, and the traffic on the commute drives her crazy. She told me that she also gets odd burning sensations in her fingertips while typing. Each night she finds that wine, which she used to drink just occasionally, is more and more compelling.

In cases like Allison's, weight loss is more about accommodating her life to her situation and finding others on her team to help with her tasks and less about starvation and boot camps.

When you feel bad and don't know why, this creates uncertainty that can raise the pressures of life even more. It is important to not ignore possibly serious symptoms, and it is also important not to feel alarmed about symptoms that do not last. If you are not sure which is which, share your concerns with your doctor.

Thankfully, you do not have to wait for the world to be perfect before you can reduce stress. To help you move from Stressed to Thriving, we can tailor your carbohydrate cycling with some additional dietary tricks. We can also repair your circadian cycles with exercise, sleep, and adaptogens; clearer thinking can be created with some easy, new breathing habits.

is it really anxiety?

Daphne was a woman in her early 30s. She was on track to move up the corporate ladder until anxiety threw her plans off course. When I asked her if there was a pattern to her anxiety, she said it was like clockwork. Each afternoon at 2:30 she feared for her life, for no apparent reason. It lasted until about 5 PM and came back at 7:30 each night. She discovered on her own that soda, juice, or alcohol would make her feel better for a few minutes, then the anxiety would come back even worse. She had been given anxiety medications by a psychiatrist but she did not like them. The medicine worked but left her too sedated to function.

When we analyzed Daphne's cortisol and blood sugar levels, we found she had a blood sugar drop each day at about 2 PM and 7 PM. Cortisol spikes came on fifteen to twenty minutes later. What was one step she could take to cure her of this frightening anxiety? Eating a breakfast with 30 grams of protein within an hour of waking up. This simple solution works because it keeps morning levels of insulin low, preventing drops in blood sugar later in the day.

your adrenals might be stressed if . . .

The most common pattern for those who are stressed is to have cortisol levels that are too high throughout the whole day (see the following chart). Note that testing is not necessary, or perfect, since cortisol is metabolized inside the fat tissue and not all of it ends up in circulation. It is best to follow your score on the Adrenal Level Quiz (Chapter 5), whether you have been tested or not.

the cure for "stressed"

The way to move from the Stressed level to that of Thriving is quite simply to reduce how much cortisol your body is making. This can happen in two main ways: by making less cortisol and by eliminating more cortisol from the body. Here, you'll find several top-rated strategies to do both and to help you lose weight easier and faster than ever before.

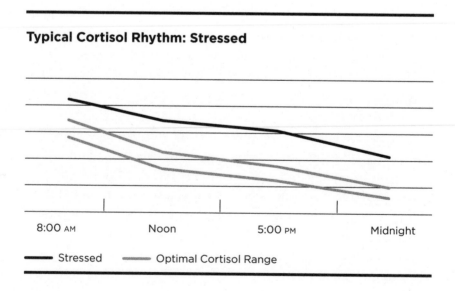

Typical Cortisol Rhythm: Stressed

8:00 AM   Noon   5:00 PM   Midnight

━━ Stressed   ━━ Optimal Cortisol Range

what to add to your ARD eating plan

Along with the general principles of the Adrenal Reset Diet (Chapter 4), there are a few more strategies that are especially helpful for those who are stressed.

reduce your sodium intake

Sodium in the diet causes the body to eliminate cortisol more slowly. Lower-salt diets help the body get rid of it faster, and that lowers the total stress level. Get in the habit of avoiding sauces in restaurants and of buying unsalted or low-salt products at the grocery store.

Keeping your total sodium intake below 3,000 mgs each day can lower all cortisol levels, food cravings, and fluid retention. But how do you know how much salt you are getting? An easy way to find out is to use a free diet-logging program. My personal favorite is My Fitness Pal, www.myfitnesspal.com.

Of the salt you do get, sea salt is good because it contains useful amounts of magnesium along with the sodium. Lite Salt is another good option; it is a brand that is much higher in potassium than regular table salt.

take a coffee break: limit caffeine to before 9 AM

Coffee and tea are popular beverages used by the majority of adults worldwide. Data has showed that both beverages may have some health benefits, such as lower risks for diabetes and Alzheimer's disease. But some people are much more prone than others to get side effects from the caffeine in these beverages, like insomnia and agitation.

Caffeine does have an effect on cortisol, but where you get your caffeine and when you have it can make all the difference. Avoiding caffeine is always an option, but not a realistic one for everyone. But if you have never lived without caffeine, you might be surprised by how calm and focused you can feel as a result. Try a two-week break from coffee or tea and afterwards make the use of caffeine a conscious choice, as opposed to a daily habit.

Another option is to switch your source of caffeine, and favor tea over coffee. Tea has caffeine like coffee, but it also has a calming compound called theanine that coffee does not have. Tea is also lower than coffee in theophylline, which stimulates the heart. For most people, consuming tea lowers their cortisol or else has little effect on it. Coffee tends not to raise your cortisol level, but it does prevent its reduction. In short, caffeine is most problematic after 9 AM. Those who are stressed can do better by limiting their coffee consumption to early in the day. Owing to the theanine, tea can be a better fit for later in the day or to assist with mental energy.

follow a low-stress diet

Along with avoiding toxic proteins and processed foods, and instituting carb cycling, you can further adjust your diet to recover from being stressed more quickly. Here are some great foods to include:

Foods that reduce cortisol production	Basil, beets, celery, cacao nibs, walnuts
Foods that replace lost nutrients due to high cortisol	Adzuki beans, almonds, kiwifruit, lemons, sweet potatoes

circadian reset and repair

move it right

Done properly, exercise can be one of the most powerful tools to break the cycle of stress and reset your Adrenal Fat Switch. With just a little strategy, it can do all of this without adding to your stress load. Studies have shown that, although any type of exercise helps, exercise done outdoors leads to greater reductions in cortisol than exercise done indoors.[1] While most of us need to move more, there are a few type As out there who can overdo it and actually harm their health through too much exercise.

Which are you? A good way to know this is by measuring your heart rate before getting out of bed. If you always train hard, take a week off and record your resting heart rate. When you resume training, keep watching it. You will know that you are overtraining when your morning resting heart rate starts to climb above where it was during your week off.

when to run and when to walk

Cortisol levels do rise for a few hours after brisk exercise of any type. Since those who are stressed are not reducing their cortisol when they should, any exercise after 2 PM should be limited to gentle yoga or walking.

cardio: less is more

As long as you are stressed, do not log hours on the treadmill. Prolonged and frequent high-intensity aerobic exercise will only make things worse. Anything above half your maximum effort will cause substantial elevations in cortisol levels. As a consequence, this will block fat loss, even though you might be burning more calories. To keep your cortisol levels in check, also avoid prolonged bouts of being sedentary.

Try wearing a pedometer or a high-tech device like a FitBit that logs your daily movement. Learn how many steps you take on average and subtract your total from 10,000. If in the course of running errands and while at work you average 6,000 steps, then plan to walk an extra 4,000 steps each day. This can be as easy as one walk of 4,000 steps or two shorter walks of 2,000 steps each. In addition to your walking, work toward spending twenty to thirty minutes in brisk aerobic activity for two days each week.

Lastly, an evening walk at a gentle pace for ten to fifteen minutes after dinner is a great way to help your prepare for sleep. It's great for your dog, too, if you have one.

strength 2.0

Strength training can do wonders to lower the survival response along with giving you other benefits, like releasing endorphins, helping the immune system, and raising metabolism. Yet it does not take large amounts of time or need to be done with much frequency to still get great results.

Plan to do two strength-training workouts each week, with movements that work the entire body. During these sessions, you can keep the cortisol from elevating by doing a gentle cardio activity like walking, jogging, or cycling for five minutes before and after your workout. Also, focus on exercises that work many different muscles at once, like old-fashioned body-weight exercises such as push-ups and jumping jacks. Visit www.adrenalresetdiet.com/resources for a free video on how to do body-weight exercises for an amazing ten-minute workout.

the home stretch

Each muscle has a bundle of nerves that control how tight it is, called *proprioceptors*. When your muscles are tight, they can make you feel tight and edgy all over. The main area of the body where tension gets built up is along back, from the neck down to the backs of the legs.

To loosen this area of tension, stand up tall, take a deep breath in, and exhale while you bend forward, reaching toward the ground with your back and knees straight. Hold the stretch for two seconds, and then bend your knees for two seconds. Repeat, straightening and bending the knees at two-second intervals for a full minute. Why the two seconds? Because your muscles start to contract and fight against a stretch after that time. By going two seconds on and two seconds off, you keep them from working against you and you loosen up much more quickly.

reset your sleep pattern

When you are stressed, sleep problems tend to be that of finding enough time for sleep and being able to get to sleep.

no time for sleep

If you cannot find enough time for sleep, this means that sleep is not yet important for you. Some of the busiest and most productive people I know manage to get 8 to 8½ hours of sleep per night. They know that it will help them get more done. But many people who are having trouble finding time to sleep simply have no idea how much better they will function with optimal amounts of it. If you are in this boat, give yourself two weeks during which you make sleep a priority, and see how much better you can feel. After trying this, most people notice that their alertness, productivity, and physical energy dramatically increase. And then sleep becomes a natural priority.

"Early to bed and early to rise" is your best strategy. If you can only justify 7½ hours for sleep, then sleeping from 10 PM to 5:30 AM will provide more benefit than sleeping from midnight to 7:30 AM. In a study of two groups of young Australians getting the same amount of sleep, those who slept later were nearly twice as likely to become obese as those who went to bed and woke up earlier.[2] Scientists think that the predators who threatened our ancestors were most active in the later parts of night. Because of this, our ancestors were able to get the deepest, most restful sleep earliest in the evening. Getting to bed no later than 10 PM can help you get more restful sleep.

can't get to sleep

If you cannot get to sleep, know that sleep aids are not the answer. Studies have shown that simple exercises and light therapy work more effectively and with no dangerous side effects. Start with progressive muscle relaxation (see page 121) for three nights. If you are still not getting seven to eight hours of quality sleep, add some light therapy (see page 122) for two weeks. Surprisingly, even those who have had decades of insomnia can often return to a good sleep rhythm with these easy steps.

say no to prescription sleep aids

Nearly 10 million American adults use prescription sleep aids most nights, and the number of regular users has been steadily rising. The most common medications include zolpidem (Ambien), eszopiclone (Lunesta), flurazepam (Dalmane), quazepam (Doral), ramelteon (Rozerem), temazepam (Restoril), triazolam (Halcion), and zaleplon (Sonata).[3]

Why not use sleep aids? Well, they are addictive, slow the brain the next day, and can make you hungrier. On average, prescription sleep aids give only a few more minutes of sleep, and it is not even high-quality sleep.

And if that is not enough reason to avoid them, know that they kill people. Regularly using sleep aids at normally prescribed dosages can raise the chance of early death by 4.5 times! But for people who are too heavy, the chances of death increase to 9 times. In a study of the use of sleep aids, "regular users" were defined as those who use them more than eighteen times per year! If you are trying to lose weight, and you use sleep aids even as infrequently as twice a month, not only are they making you groggier and less able to lose weight but they are putting your life in jeopardy.[4]

Why are sleeping pills hard to quit taking? Most people who try to quit suffer rebound insomnia. This means that when they stop taking the medication, their sleep is even worse than before. If you are hooked on sleep aids, use the relaxation tips on page 121 to improve your sleep patterns and work with your doctor to establish a safe withdrawal schedule. (With your doctor's help, you can do this with the Wake Therapy protocol in Chapter 7, page 141.)

reprogram with progressive muscle relaxation

What happens to a kid when he gets bored in school? He becomes restless and can't sit still. But after playing at recess, he is again able to sit and regain focus. As adults we also build up nervous tension as the day goes on; unfortunately, most of us don't have recess time to "play it out." If you find yourself in bed and unable to shut off your brain, nervous tension may be the culprit. Here's a simple technique that can reverse this nervous tension. It has also been shown to work better than medications for falling asleep faster and staying asleep longer. The technique is called progressive muscle relaxation, or PMR for short.

You start out by lying on your back in bed. Move around if you need to, and adjust the sheets or covers to get comfortable. Once you are settled in, begin alternating deep breathing with holding your breath and squeezing your muscles. This is done in steps, working your way through all the muscle groups of the body. Start with your toes and feet, and work your way up. Here it is, in four easy steps:

Step 1. Take a deep breath in and hold it for a slow count of 5. As you are holding your breath, contract your toes and the muscles of your feet as tightly as you can.

Step 2. After the count of 5, exhale and immediately release all the tension in your toes and feet.

Step 3. Take three slow breaths and feel the relaxation in your feet. If they still feel somewhat tense, repeat the first two steps one or two more times.

Step 4: After the feet, work upward, muscle by muscle. Next up is your calves, then your thighs, followed by your hips, your abdomen and torso, your arms, and finally your head, neck, and face. (It is common to need an extra cycle or two to get all the tension out of your head and neck area.)

The average response to PMR is that a person falls asleep twenty minutes faster and gains thirty to ninety minutes of quality sleep.

PMR has also been shown to improve immune function and reset cortisol metabolism.[5]

shedding a little light on light therapy

Part of the reason many of us have sleep problems is that we no longer wake up at sunrise and go to sleep soon after sunset. Our brains control our sleep cycle based on the rhythm of sunlight and darkness, but artificial light and light pollution disrupt this cycle. Light therapy can do wonders in helping regulating your whole day's cortisol response and getting more sleep, and this can be done in nature or with light boxes.

The ideal exposure to help your reset is to gain thirty minutes of bright overhead light exposure during the first hour of being awake. For example, on sunny days, take a nice walk or have a leisurely breakfast outside. On days when the sun or your schedule does not cooperate, use a light box overhead—perhaps while you have your breakfast shake and make plans for the day. If you are totally time-crunched, you can even do some computer work under the light box and gain the same effects. As your sleep improves, you can reduce the light exposure time by five minutes per day, down to a maintenance dose of fifteen minutes.

 ## adrenal tonics for the stressed

Those who are stressed can improve their health and weight-loss efforts by using nonprescription supplements to speed their cortisol recovery. These supplements can help the stressed to move toward thriving in as little as a few weeks rather than a few months.

Unfortunately, many adrenal formulas contain ingredients that are not a good fit for this stage, such as rhodiola, or 5HTP. Other common ingredients to avoid if you are stressed include licorice root or adrenal cortex extracts, as they can raise cortisol rather than lower it. The other pitfall is that many remedies used to lower cortisol are too sedating for daytime use. However, here are a couple of safe and effective suggestions.

morning adrenal tonic: lemon balm

In a double blind study of humans, lemon balm (*Melissa officiana-lis*) has been shown to achieve the nearly impossible. It can both reduce the effect of stress and increase alertness, with no significant risks or side effects. Compared to a control group taking a placebo, those using lemon balm felt calmer when challenged by stress and they also did better on math tests.[6] What is there not to love?

Lemon balm is an herb that is readily available in powder form in most health food stores, and it's easy to grow in a home garden. It is not an expensive supplement, and it works well at dosages as low as 25 to 50 mg.[7] Magnesium and a Chinese herb called *scutellaria* work well with lemon balm to help enhance its cortisol-reducing effects. Along with being a supplement, lemon balm makes a tasty tea and can readily be found in tea bags.

evening adrenal tonic: magnolia bark and passionflower

Magnolia bark (*Magnolia officianalis*) has been used for thousands of years in Chinese medicine as a gentle sedative to reduce anxiety and pain. Today we know that it contains a compound called honokiol, which works like anxiety medicines but much more safely.

Benzodiazepine medicines such as Ativan, Xanax, and Valium can reduce anxiety and help people fall asleep. They are dangerously addictive, however, and can lead to early dementia when used for as little as several months.[8] A plant called passionflower works in the same ways as benzodiazepine medications, but without their addictive and brain-damaging properties.[9]

Passionflower is most effective when standardized to contain 3.5 percent flavonoids, and it can safely be used as needed or on a regular basis, in pill form or as tea. Most effective doses range from 33 to 66 mg.[10] Passionflower extracts are available without a prescription in health food stores; however, those on prescription sleep or mood medications should use it only with medical supervision.

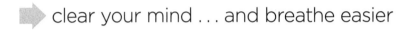 clear your mind . . . and breathe easier

When you are stressed, there are real problems that demand your attention. These can include financial demands, health concerns, and family matters. Alas, they are matters you really cannot just ignore or avoid. The good news is that by improving your mental state, you can take care of them even better. Spending as little as a few minutes doing the breathing techniques below can produce results that are life-changing for both you and those around you.

morning habit: alternate nostril breathing

Did you know that you breathe out of one nostril more than the other in a rhythm that alternates throughout the day? This is called the *nasal cycle*. The duration for each nostril varies from forty minutes to a few hours. Although scientists have been aware of this cycle, it is just recently that its purpose has been discovered.

Some chemicals that we smell are better detected by the fast-moving air of the dominant nostril. Others chemicals are best picked up by the slow-moving air of the resting nostril. By switching back and forth, these nerves stay fresh. Since this cycle is regulated by the part of the brain that also controls our fight-or-flight response, it becomes disrupted when we are stressed. By intentionally controlling which nostril receives air for how long, you can quickly reset the system and lower your level of stress.

The basic idea is to alternate which nostril you breathe through. Sit in a comfortable position with your back straight. Use a tissue to clear your sinuses, if needed. Each step should be done while slowly counting to 4.

Step 1: Breathe in through your right nostril.

Step 2: Close both nostrils and hold.

Step 3: Exhale from your left nostril.

Step 4: Inhale from your left nostril.

Step 5: Hold your breath for a count, closing both nostrils.

Step 6: Exhale from your right nostril.

Those steps make one cycle. Repeat the cycles for a total of five minutes. As you practice, you will find that your breathing becomes slower. When this happens, move the count to a higher number. Alternate nostril breathing is best done within one hour of waking, so as to help reset the circadian cycle.

anytime vacation: diaphragmatic breathing

Our bodies are engineered to breathe deeply by moving our abdomens in and out. When we are in survival mode, we breathe quickly and more shallowly. Depending on whether your brain is surviving or thriving, your body will act accordingly. Thankfully this works both ways; by consciously coaxing your body to act as it does when thriving, your brain follows suit.

For this reason, breathing deep from the diaphragm reverses the effects of stress and stimulates the flow of lymphatic fluid throughout the body. Beneficial effects can be felt in as little as a few seconds, or a few breaths, with this practice.

Diaphragmatic breathing can be done most effectively when standing, but it also can be done while sitting. It can even be done inconspicuously without disrupting co-workers. Restroom breaks can be an easy time to practice.

TO BEGIN: The first few times you do the exercise, place your right palm on your stomach directly over your belly button. This can be done over clothing. Breathe in deeply with the intention of moving your hand out with your inhalation and letting it move back in as you exhale. You should clearly see your hand move several inches when you're doing it properly. It is also common to feel your clothes more snugly against your abdomen at the deepest part of the inhalation.

TO CONTINUE: During the practice sessions, close your eyes and slowly inhale through your mouth as you expand your abdomen as much as possible. Focus on feeling your breath move into your body and fill your abdomen. After completely inhaling, slowly exhale though your mouth as you pull your abdomen in as tight as you can. Plan for three breaths for a quick refresh or ten breaths for a thorough reset anytime you need it.

a sample day for the stressed

Here is a quick primer on how these techniques can easily fit into the busiest of schedules.

WAKE UP

Thirty minutes of bright light within the first hour

BREAKFAST

ARD high-protein breakfast

Morning walk, or 20 minutes of strength or cardio training

MORNING ROUTINES

Alternate nostril breathing for 5 minutes

Lemon balm tea

LUNCH

ARD balanced lunch

ANYTIME VACATION

Diaphragmatic breathing, 3 to 10 breaths

DINNER

ARD healthy carb dinner

BEDTIME RITUALS

Progressive muscle relaxation

Passionflower tea

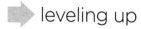 leveling up

Moving off of the Stressed level and up to the Thriving level is within your reach and clearly possible. Even if life's stressors are substantial, you can improve your health by using the Adrenal Reset Diet and tips from this chapter. Retake your Adrenal Level Quiz each month. It is good to take the quiz on the first day of each month, to make sure you are moving in the right direction. Starting from the first day, your health will improve and stress will have less of an effect on your weight.

Most people find that by following the ADR, improving their sleep patterns, and devoting just a few minutes each day to breathing exercises, they can be at the Thriving level within two to four weeks.

wired and tired

WHEN PEOPLE ARE WIRED AND TIRED, THE CORE ISSUE IS THAT their adrenal hormone levels are highly variable. Rather than having a consistent morning peak and evening shut-off, people at this level can make too much cortisol late in the day and too much early in the day. This often causes their energy levels to be erratic and inconsistent. They will often have brief peaks of great clarity and productivity, separated by longer bouts of fatigue and mental fog. Often, people who are at the Wired and Tired level can predict that some times of day will be better or worse than others. For example, they may know that they always crash in the afternoon and get a burst of energy around bedtime. It is also common for people at this level to be aware of unstable blood sugar levels. They may feel very frantic or edgy if a meal is delayed or missed.

Being Wired and Tired is a state that usually develops after several months of substantial stressors. These stressors could be significant changes to health, challenges like an illness or death of a loved one, or layoff threats at work. There are many people who get to this level, though, from less obvious stressors that add up over longer periods of time, such as many years of poor food choices or poor sleep habits.

The main shift in the adrenal system when moving to a state of

Wired and Tired is that the daily cycle starts to erode. Morning levels of cortisol may be lower and nighttime levels may be higher. The difference between the two is called the *cortisol slope*. You can think of this relationship just like a ski slope. When the slope is steep, the skiing is good. Without a slope, you would not have much fun.

How important is the cortisol slope? In a study in Britain that was run from 2002 to 2004, over 4,000 adults were evaluated for longevity factors, including age, weight, gender, tobacco use, sleep habits, blood sugar levels, history of heart disease, and exercise. They were also given tests to see how steep their cortisol slopes were.

When all was said and done, the strongest predictor of early death was the lack of a cortisol slope (see Table 7.1). It was a stronger predictor than even whether people smoked or how overweight they were.[1]

I have shared the results of this study with many patients who have dismissed the importance of slowing down and managing stress. Many people who would never jeopardize their health by smoking do not realize that, by straining their adrenal glands, they are facing even greater risks.

TABLE 7.1. WHITEHALL II STUDY: TOTAL DEATHS AND CAUSES

CAUSE OF DEATH	TOTAL DEATHS
Abnormal cortisol slope	138
Smoking	136
Obesity	133

rachel's story: an insider's look at "wired and tired"

Rachel was an attorney in her mid-30s who was at her wit's end. Along with her weight being a source of stress, her career was on the line. After recently getting a good position in a large firm, she was in danger of losing it because her performance was declining. Her career would live or die based on how many billable hours she produced. Yet, owing to her declining memory and failing powers of concentration, fewer partners in the firm were confident enough to refer clients to her.

Rachel finished near the top of her class, but knew that the pace of law school had taken a toll on her. She had justified it by telling herself she would relax more after school was over. Of course, the years following were far from relaxing. Her weight had not been ideal since high school, but she always had been able to stay within 10 pounds of her goal by exercising enough. After the first few years in practice, three things seemed to happen at the same time: her weight went up by 6 or 7 pounds a year, her sleep had gradually deteriorated, and her short-term memory had gotten worse. She was also too fatigued to do any significant amount of exercise.

I taught Rachel about carbohydrate cycling and I insisted she take weekends and evenings off from work. She was concerned that doing so would cause her to fall further behind. Within the first few weeks, however, her productivity started going up even though she was working fewer hours. Her weight began to come down, although slowly at first. As her energy came back, she was confident resuming exercise would help the rest of it come off faster.

what happens when you're wired and tired

How does being Wired and Tired affect your health? Imagine a car pulling a trailer up a long, steep road. When you are thriving, the stressors come and go but they don't cause you to lose your momentum. The car is running cool and maintaining speed just fine. This is what in our bodies would be called *healthy compensation*. When you are stressed, however, there has been too much on your plate for a while; your adrenal system is working overtime to see you through it. The car is still managing to maintain its speed uphill, but the engine is working hard and heating up. You can think of this as *overcompensation*.

When you reach the Wired and Tired stage, it all starts to change drastically. Now the car is starting to sputter and lose speed. There are also some warning lights on the dash. This is the first stage of *decompensation*; the system is starting to not function right.

your adrenals might be wired and tired if . . .

The most common cortisol pattern for those who are Wired and Tired is a daily curve in reverse: lower levels of cortisol in the morning and higher levels in the evening. Overall, the amount of cortisol made is healthy, but it is made at the wrong times. Again, note that testing is not a perfect view into your cortisol levels, since cortisol is metabolized inside the fat tissue and not all of it ends up in circulation. Here, as with other levels, it is best to follow your score on the Adrenal Level Quiz (Chapter 5).

Typical Cortisol Rhythm: Wired and Tired

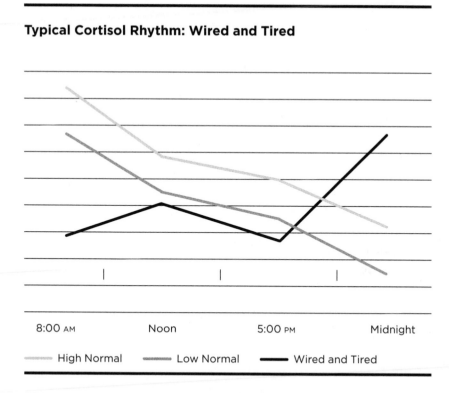

| 8:00 AM | Noon | 5:00 PM | Midnight |

······ High Normal   ▬▬▬ Low Normal   ▬▬▬ Wired and Tired

▶ the cure for wired and tired

As tough as it is to be Wired and Tired, this is one of the quickest states to recover from. Stress hormones are being made; there is usually not too many or too few of them, it is just that they are being made at the wrong times of the day. By following the ARD, and using the tricks below to help reset your circadian rhythm, you can be back to thriving in one to three weeks.

An important principle to keep in mind with Wired and Tired is that the schedule is everything. Those who have managed babies know that with precise timing of food, sleep, and activity, life is good. Throw off the routine, though, and everything falls apart. Grown-ups who are Wired and Tired have the exact same needs. When you eat and sleep is just as important as what you eat and how much you sleep.

⇒ what to add to your ARD eating plan

Those who are Wired and Tired benefit from a few extra dietary strategies to reset their daily rhythms so that they can have an easier time losing weight. In many cases, those at this level are not hungry for breakfast, but they get ravenous in the evening and end up bingeing on salty or sweet foods like chips, ice cream, cookies, or pretzels. Having a good breakfast with 25 to 30 grams of complete protein can help change this in as little as three to eight days. Soon the evening appetite calms down and hunger itself starts to work as an alarm clock.

For those who are Wired and Tired, gentle culinary spices can also be useful for resetting their rhythms. Two of the best are ginger and cinnamon.

ginger

Entire books have been written about the health benefits of ginger. Along with reducing inflammation and improving circulation, ginger has been shown to lower the response to stress from both the adrenals and the pituitary gland.[2] Ginger is versatile and can be used in a variety of forms. Powdered ginger and grated fresh ginger are both effective. Companies even make frozen ginger with removable individual, serving-sized containers. (These are my favorite since they have the convenience of dried ginger but the taste of fresh.) Ginger can be added to protein shakes, hot cereals, soups, and cooked dishes. For ginger tea, 1 to 2 teaspoons of fresh ginger or 1/2 to 1 teaspoon of dried is enough to improve the stress response.

cinnamon

A kitchen staple with adrenal-healing powers is cinnamon. Specifically, cinnamon has been shown to help reset the Adrenal Fat Switch when insomnia throws it into storage mode.[3]

The vicious cycle that dominates the Wired and Tired stage is that lack of sleep makes the muscles send blood sugar to the fat tissue. This promotes fat growth as more calories go in to the fat tissue and it makes the adrenals work harder to control the blood sugar. As little as ½ teaspoon ground cinnamon each day can help with this. Cinnamon is added easily to hot cereals, teas, and dishes with meat or poultry. I don't encourage using cinnamon in capsule form. In this state, a large amount is released in a small area of the esophagus or the stomach and can cause significant irritation or burning, especially if a capsule gets stuck when swallowing.

other foods for the wired and tired

Here are a few more foods you can eat that will help get your daily rhythms back to normal.

Foods that regulate cortisol	Whole grain barley, white beans, cabbage, Brazil nuts
Foods that help replace nutrients lost from erratic cortisol	Bok choy, spinach, oysters, pumpkin seeds

circadian reset and repair

move it right

Along with the right type, duration, and intensity of exercise, its timing is also critical to help reset the daily rhythm of your adrenal glands. Getting up early and being outside in the morning sun will be much more beneficial than hitting the gym on the way home from work. Try to only do strenuous exercise earlier in the day, so as to not further disrupt the afternoon and evening cortisol levels. Gentle yoga or walking can be fine for afternoon or evening activities.

cardio conditioning—HIT the road

Timed right, high-intensity interval training can be especially helpful. Twice weekly do a morning interval workout while running outdoors or on any aerobic machine. Warm up for five minutes, then start doing intervals. The intervals should consist of thirty- to sixty-second bursts at your highest intensity, followed by one- to two-minute cycles at an easy pace. After five intervals, do a five-minute cooldown and you're all done!

strength 2.0

Plan to do strength training for your whole body twice weekly for twenty to thirty minutes each session. Complex movements that involve multiple joints are the most helpful because they stimulate nerves that reset your daily rhythms. These movements include squatting, lunging, lifting, balancing, and rotating. Give yourself one to two minutes between each exercise and do ten minutes of low-intensity cardio, like walking or jogging, at the end of your workout.

the home stretch

Soothing stretching sessions of three minutes, done an hour before bed, are helpful for lowering the evening's cortisol levels. Yoga poses that invert your body and get your legs above your head are most helpful. A simple pose that works well is called the shoulder stand.

To do the shoulder stand, lie on your back and bring your legs over your head. Next, use your hands to support your hips as you raise your legs above you. (If that is challenging, you can also lie with your hips against a wall and rest your legs against the wall.) Hold the position and breathe deeply.

reset your sleep pattern

when you only get tired at the wrong times

People who are Wired and Tired often can sleep, but not at practical times. They may notice that after a night of tossing and turning, they finally go into a deep sleep at 4 or 5 AM. If possible, they would happily stay up until early morning and sleep until late in the day. Usually, most life schedules will not accommodate this. Many struggle with trying to go to bed earlier, but find that it just does not work. Although it is nearly impossible to move your sleep cycle to an earlier time, most people can stay up four hours later and sleep four hours later with little problem. If this is done for a few days over a long weekend, the sleep schedule can be completely repaired.

How does this work? Imagine that someone regularly cannot not fall asleep until 4 AM, but she needs to wake for work at 6 AM each day, and she would like to sleep for over seven hours. Here is how she can reset her body's circadian rhythm in five days. Note that this works best when sleeping in as much darkness as possible and waking up to the brightest light possible.

Day 1: Stay awake 24 hours, until an 8 AM bedtime, then wake up at 3 PM.

Day 2: Bedtime at noon, wake up at 7 PM.

Day 3: Bedtime at 4 PM, wake up at 11 PM.

Day 4: Bedtime at 8 PM, wake up at 3 AM.

Day 5: Bedtime 11 PM, wake up at 6 AM.

shedding a little light on light therapy

Light therapy is another trick that can be helpful for moving your schedule back to normal. Since many people at this level find themselves falling asleep too late, light therapy has to be done differently than for those at the Stressed level. Rather than first thing in the morning, use thirty minutes of bright overhead light exposure in the early evening—ideally, five hours before your projected bedtime.

For most people this is not possible with sunlight. For this trick to work well, you also need to *avoid* bright light for the first few hours of the morning during the first two weeks of light therapy. This is done by staying indoors until two hours after waking and by wearing dark glasses if you must go out for a commute to work.

blueblockers to the rescue

We mark our days by the rising and the setting of the sun. Throughout the day, the sun gives color in the full spectrum: red, orange, yellow, green, blue, indigo, and violet. As the sun sets, the shorter wavelengths of blue, indigo, and violet become blocked, all light is more scattered and indirect, and all shadows disappear. Things take on more vivid hues of red, orange, and yellow. This is why photographers call the last hour of the day the "golden hour."

Our daily cycles of waking and sleeping are strongly controlled by these same color changes. Yet most artificial light has more of the blue wavelengths than natural light does during any time of day. This is especially true for computers, televisions, and display screens. This extra blue light exposure is thought to be behind the increasing rates of both insomnia and some cancers like colon cancer.[4]

f.lux is a free program you can download that adjusts your computer's color output to fit the time of day for your location. It works on both a Mac and a PC, and should be available soon for mobile devices. For artificial lights you cannot control, there are glasses like Uvex that can help. Wear them starting an hour before bed, and they can block most environmental blue light and help improve your sleep.

Please note that as good as this trick is for a reset, it is not a long-term strategy. Morning sunlight is a pleasure not to be denied when your rhythms are reset. As your sleep improves, resume normal morning light exposure. If your sleep ever slips back to where you wake too early, move your light exposure back to the evening again.

wake therapy

For those with the very worst insomnia, here are the big guns for sleep repair! The process typically takes four to eight days and can work in even the toughest of cases. The first few of these days you may be even more tired than normal. Don't plan to do these first days when you are giving that make-or-break presentation or are getting ready for final exams.

To start, it is helpful to estimate how many of hours of sleep you currently are getting, even if they are broken up. For example, if you fall asleep at 11:30 PM, wake up at 2 AM, cannot get back to sleep until 3 AM, and then wake for good at 5 AM, this would be considered 4½ hours of total sleep. We use this number in planning the therapy.

Next, decide on your ideal time to wake up. Consider your school and/or work schedules, family duties, and the best time to start the day if sleep were not an issue. We will use 6 AM for the purposes of this example. The general plan, then, is that sleep is restricted to the number of hours you currently get, ending at your wake-up time. You want to avoid sleeping at any other times of the day. Gradually, the scheduled sleep times are expanded. Your rhythms are reset because your body gets so tired the first few nights that you cannot help but fall asleep. Once you have fully reset your rhythms, good sleep is automatic. Here is how it works.

Let's say you get 4½ hours of sleep on your own and you'd like to wake up at 6 AM. On the first day, you stay awake until 4½ hours before 6 AM, or 1:30 AM. At 6 AM, you wake up, using multiple alarm clocks if needed. Immediately after waking, you let your body know that this is morning; you can do this by being outside in bright lights, moving in some way, and being around people. A quick trip to a coffee shop can be an effective (and needed!) way to get out and about. During that whole first day, you want to do whatever you can to avoid napping. The next evening, you add fifteen minutes to your sleep time without changing what time you wake up. In this example, that would mean going to bed at 1:15 AM. Again, you wake up, be active, and stay awake all day until bedtime. Each night you go to bed fifteen minutes earlier. You continue this process until you are satisfied with your sleep.

The vast majority of those with longstanding insomnia can regain healthy sleep by following this process carefully. The therapy is so powerful that many also use it to help break away from sleep aids. Of course, you want support and assistance from your doctor if you plan to do this.

adrenal tonics for the wired and tired

The goal is not to lower or raise cortisol, but to help the body make the right amounts at the right times. One of the most useful tonics for this stage is ashwaganda (*Withania somnifera*).

morning adrenal tonic: a rose by any other name

Rhodiola (*Rhodiola rosea*) is also known as rose root; it is the best fit when stress leads to fatigue, anxiety, and a lack of mental focus. The versions that worked in the studies were standardized extracts. Rhodiola is available from most pharmacies, health food stores, or online supplement retailers. Look at the label for 0.8 to 1.0 percent salidroside and 2 to 4 percent rosavin. Most who use rhodiola experience the benefits with as little as 100 to 300 mg daily. Since a small percentage of people may feel stimulated by it, it is best taken in the morning.[5, 6]

evening adrenal tonic: ashwaganda

Ashwaganda is a Sanskrit word meaning "smells like a horse." Don't let the name put you off; ashwaganda has some serious "horsepower" when it comes to fixing your adrenals. It is unique among supplements in that it eases anxiety symptoms and can protect brain cells from the damages of stress. Many tonics can act as stimulants, but not this one. Overstimulation is a problem if you are Wired and

Tired, but this long-used tonic aims to calm. The many documented benefits of ashwaganda include:

- Helping immune function
- Improving memory and learning
- Stabilizing blood sugar
- Reducing stress-induced damage to brain cells

Since ashwaganda helps correct cortisol levels, it can be a good fit for boosting morning energy levels and lowering them at night. A normal dose is 500 to 1,000 mg once or twice daily of the powdered root in capsules. Please note that ashwaganda may also influence thyroid function, usually in a good way. Those on thyroid replacement should regularly test their blood levels if taking ashwaganda in case they need a reduction in dosage.[7]

 clear your mind . . . and regain focus

When people are Wired and Tired, their mental state can be greatly upset. Along with being unpleasant, worrisome thoughts and anxiety can become causes of higher levels of stress in their own right. Learning to calm the mind and break this vicious cycle of stress is one of the most powerful ways to reset your rhythms and it is ridiculously simple!

the relaxation response

Today we take it for granted that blood pressure levels can be higher in a doctor's office than they are at home. There is even an official name for it: white-coat hypertension. But just a few decades ago, medical professionals did not believe that the mind could affect the body in ways like this. As late as 1969, Dr. Herbert Benson proved that stress like bright lights could raise the blood pressure of monkeys. His work gained the attention of the new Transcendental

Meditation community, pioneered by Maharishi Mahesh Yogi, the famous guru to the Beatles.

Advanced meditators believed that they could control their blood pressure levels at will and they wanted someone like Dr. Benson to prove this to the world. His studies bore out their claims, and also showed that meditators were less apt to get stuck in survival mode.

Dr. Benson saw clear benefits to meditation, but also saw barriers that would prevent it from being used by many who could be well served by it. The methods were complicated and took years to learn. They also involved rituals and concepts that some might feel went against their religious practices. Dr. Benson set out to find a simple and nondenominational technique that still would be effective. With his work, he showed that most of the benefits of meditation could come with as little as a five-minute session once to twice daily, using a practice he called the *relaxation response*. Anyone can learn it in a few minutes and experience immediate benefits. The technique became the focus of many later studies, all proving its effectiveness. Here's how to trigger it.

TO BEGIN: Choose a time and place where you will be comfortable and will not be interrupted. You want to be cozy enough to relax but not enough to fall asleep. Sitting upright in a chair works best for most people. Decide on the duration of your practice and set a timer with a gentle tone. Choose a focus word you find peaceful and relaxing. This can be a name or concept from your religious tradition or something more universal like love or peace.

NEXT: Close your eyes and consciously relax the muscles from your feet to your head for about a minute. Breathe slowly and repeat your focus word as you exhale. Expect your mind to wander and expect to lose track of what you're doing, especially at first. Once you catch yourself wandering, simply restore your attention to your focus word and your breathing. When your timer sounds, take an unstructured minute or so to ready yourself to get up and resume your activities.

high-tech solutions for lazy meditators

Sound-light Machines

Have you ever heard a catchy rhythm and had it stick in your head? Even at an unconscious level, the human brain mimics patterns. Whether you are awake, alert, dreamy, or asleep is a function of the rate of pulsations of your brain waves. When you see lights or hear sounds that pulse in certain frequencies, your brain waves mimic those frequencies. During meditation, the brain goes into what is called an *alpha state.* Machines are available that create pulses of light and sound to get the brain to shift its waves to a targeted state. These work with specially made goggles and headphones, and can immediately produce the effects of advanced meditation. Look to the resources section for information on specific sound-light machines.

Just Beat It

Binaural beats are not the latest high-fashion headphones; rather, they are the same idea as light and sound therapy, but without the light. All you need is a way to play music and a pair of headphones. Because specific sounds go to each side of the headphone or ear buds, these do not work without headphones. There are also downloadable MP3 files that allow you to use your music player or smartphone to produce binaural beats through a headset. My favorite is called Brainwave, and it has binaural programs for everything from waking up, critical thinking, and enhancing exercise to helping induce sleep.

a sample day for the wired and tired

Here is a quick primer on how these techniques can easily fit into the busiest of schedules.

WAKE UP

30 minutes of bright light 2 hours after waking

BREAKFAST

ARD high-protein breakfast

Rhodiola tonic

MORNING ROUTINES

Morning walk or interval training

Relaxation response for 5 minutes

LUNCH

ARD balanced lunch

ANYTIME VACATION

Listen to binaural beats while doing other activities

DINNER

ARD healthy-carb dinner

BEDTIME RITUALS

Wake therapy (short-term reset)

Take ashwaganda

leveling up

Moving from the Wired and Tired level can happen promptly when the circumstances are right. Those who focus on the Adrenal Reset Diet and take five to ten minutes a day to lower their load of physical stress often find that they can move back to the Thriving level within one to three weeks. It is good to repeat your Adrenal Level Quiz (Chapter 5) on the first day of each month to make sure you are moving in the right direction and staying on track.

crashed

HOW DOES IT FEEL TO CRASH? NOT GOOD, THAT IS FOR SURE. Crashed is the most severe dysfunction of the adrenal system. In it, the body is trying to protect itself by going into a state of forced hibernation. Whether you call this "adrenal collapse," "blowing out your adrenals," or an "adrenal crisis," one thing is for sure—it is not fun. What is happening is that the body has been under so many cumulative stressors from the pressures of life, processed foods, and pollutants that cortisol production has been decreased to prevent further damage. Note that cortisol is being reduced not because it cannot be made; it is because the demands of high cortisol cannot be tolerated. This is why simply taking cortisol as a medicine is not helpful for those who are at the Crashed level.

My grandfather had one of the larger farm trucks in our neck of the woods in northern Minnesota, and it was also one of the oldest. He named it "Methuselah" in reference to the 900+-year-old character in the Bible. His biggest fear was that the engine would fail on a distant field and it would be a nightmare to get it out. To protect the old engine so it would not die in the wrong place, Grandpa put a block of wood under the gas pedal so no one could give it too much throttle. When you are Crashed, this is what is happening. Your body has placed a block of wood under your gas pedal so you are forced to slow down.

If your Adrenal Level Quiz (Chapter 5) led you to this chapter, it is important to be tested and examined by a skilled doctor to rule out other medical conditions. I believe that everyone deserves TLC and regular medical care to make sure there are no problems lurking, but this is doubly true if you are Crashed. I cannot overemphasize this point.

Many people have come to me assuming that their symptoms were all the consequences of stress, poor sleep, or bad habits, only to find out that there were medical issues that had not yet been diagnosed. Here are just a few of the more common ones you would want to be checked for:

- Thyroid disease

- Anemia

- Diabetes / hypoglycemia

- Chronic Epstein-Barr virus

- Kidney disease

- Heart disease

- Fatty liver disease

- Sick building syndrome

- Nutrient deficiencies

- Sleep apnea

 ## what happens when you're crashed

Those who find themselves in a Crashed state have often led up to it with long periods of multiple demands and pressures. These are often multiple major life events like illnesses, care of loved ones, or financial pressures that have drawn out for many years. In addition, some who are Crashed have a personality type of being eager to please or help others. They may have a hard time saying no when asked to contribute. In any event, they find themselves overextended for too long. To heal your adrenals, you need less on your plate and more time to care for yourself.

suzanne's story: an insider's look at "crashed"

"The last few years seem to have dragged on forever. I feel like I've been walking through molasses. Everything I do is hard and doesn't seem to be worth the effort."

Suzanne was only in her early 30s when she told me this. Her main reason for seeing me was a stubborn 15 pounds she could not shake. But after speaking for just a few minutes, she confided in me what was really going on. She was a health-care practitioner herself, and her health was collapsing under her workload. Between 60+ hour workweeks and poor sleep, she developed a number of chronic respiratory infections that medications could not seem to cure.

The more tired Suzanne got, the more behind she was on her workload. She had not participated in social activities for years. Any limited time off was spent sleeping and trying to regain her energy. She was under my care for thyroid disease, but she checked in so rarely that I had not known how bad things had gotten. Once she explained what was going on, I did comprehensive tests, including for her adrenal function. It turned out that her cortisol levels were so low that she needed to get a medic alert bracelet, as it would be critical knowledge for any unforeseen emergency medical care.

I carefully explained to her how serious her situation was, and I helped her realize that her health had to become her top priority for the next few months. I encouraged her to cut her workload in half and spend ten days on the beach, with no schedule or obligations. This was a perfect setting to jump into the ARD. Over the months that followed she took targeted supplements and participated in acupuncture and regular meditation. Six months later, she was so pleased with her increased energy and mood that she did not even mention her weight loss until I brought it up. She was noticeably fitter and back down to her ideal weight again.

your adrenals might be crashed if ...

The core feature of being Crashed is the overwhelming exhaustion. Common symptoms include debilitating fatigue, muscle wasting, mid-body obesity, a feeling of general weakness, cravings for sugar or salt, and dizziness when getting up suddenly. There can also be muscle aches and pains, joint pain, unusually low blood pressure, and a variety of digestive symptoms including gas and bloating.

Because those who are at this level have a hard time being physically active and interacting with others, they are at substantial risk for major depression and weight gain, as well as at increased risk of heart disease and diabetes. If that's you, improving your health needs to be your the main priority.

The most common cortisol pattern for those who are Crashed is levels that are below target throughout the whole day. Again,

Typical Cortisol Rhythm: Crashed

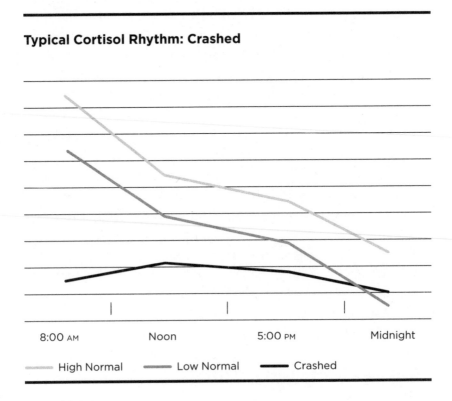

| 8:00 AM | Noon | 5:00 PM | Midnight |

High Normal — Low Normal — Crashed

testing is not perfect, since cortisol is metabolized inside the fat tissue and not all of it ends up in circulation. It is best to follow your score on the Adrenal Level Quiz (Chapter 5), even if your test results differ.

 ## the cure for crashed

When someone is Crashed, he or she can heal and start to notice benefits within days of taking the right steps. Full recovery is possible in rarely more than six to eight weeks when health is made a top priority.

the priorities game: what really matters?

Often, people have a hard time justifying a needed reduction in activities. What is really worthy of your time? Here is a revealing game that will help you learn your priorities. Find a piece of paper, a pen or pencil, and about ten minutes to think.

> *Step 1*: Sit down and write down a list of your top-ten time commitments. Think of any extra things you do for work, on social media, with outside clubs or organizations you assist, or charities, activities, or social obligations. Write down the first ten that come to mind.

> *Step 2*: Imagine that whomever is closest to you just had a health scare. You know for sure the person will be fine, but he needs you by his side for two hours per day for the next two months. Which seven obligations could you cross off your list to be there?

> *Step 3:* Most of us would do more for a loved one than we would for ourselves. Instead of crossing off seven obligations, cross five off your original list. You have just cut half of your obligations and freed up two hours per day for rest and personal care. At the level of being Crashed, your health is that critical.

just say no

Remember the anti-drug campaign from the 1980s? To move out of Crashed and back toward Thriving takes discipline. You need to reduce your activities to those that are most essential and say no to all the rest. This is a time when it is worthwhile to call in any favors and rely heavily on friends and family. If managed well, you can come away from this with a renewed sense of perspective and priorities. If managed poorly, though, this can be a slippery slope toward a narrowing envelope of capabilities and a growing list of medical issues to deal with long term.

 ## what to add to your ARD eating plan

It is possible to lose weight when you are Crashed, but it is important to be gentle and give yourself time. At this level, even taking on positive changes can feel overwhelming. Your energy levels will be more stable with more frequent meals. Since it is hard for your adrenals to make enough cortisol, your blood sugar can easily and quickly drop off. When this happens, it jolts your already tired adrenals to work even harder.

Even though you need to keep your blood sugar up, remember that foods that raise your blood sugar the quickest also make it drop off the worst. Your best bets are the protein shakes and healthy meals of ARD on a regular schedule and having snacks from the unlimited food list regularly, both mid-morning and mid-afternoon.

special foods for the crashed

There are some foods that can specifically aid in your recovery. Include these several times per week and watch how quickly your energy comes back.

Foods that help low cortisol	Grapefruit, maca, sesame seeds, tumeric
Foods with nutrients needed owing to low cortisol levels	Avocado, grass-fed beef, sea salt

increase your sodium intake

Let your body make more use of the cortisol it has; sodium causes cortisol to stay in your system longer. And although extra salt is not helpful for other levels of adrenal stress, those who are Crashed often have very low blood pressure, so a little extra salt can help them regain energy. This should be thought of as a short-term remedy for the six to eight weeks of recovery, since the data shows that too much salt poses a danger, even for those with low blood pressure.[1]

 # circadian reset and repair

We have learned that these daily cycles are vital for health and weight loss. In the case of Crashed, when the circadian cycle is repaired, energy levels pick up, mood symptoms get better, and the body's ability to lose weight comes back online. Along with the ARD, the tips here will get your daily rhythms and quality sleep back in no time.

move it right

EASY DOES IT

At this level, too much exercise can easily do more harm than good. Do not pressure yourself into thinking that you need regular, structured, strenuous activity. A gentle morning walk in the sun for ten to twenty minutes is ideal. Time spent gently moving in water that is close to body temperature is also therapeutic. When cortisol levels are chronically low, the individual fibers of muscle tissue tend to become less mobile and easily stick together. This creates pain and immobility, which raises stress and further drives the survival response. Regular massage and use of a foam roller on any tender spots can help this dramatically.

IF YOU ARE NEW TO EXERCISE

If you do not exercise and do not enjoy it, start with a ten- to twenty-minute morning walk. After a few weeks of this, consider adding a second walk to your evening routines. The National Weight Loss Registry has been tracking those who have successfully kept significant amounts of weight off for several years. One of the few common threads has been a total walking distance of 4 miles daily. Once you get a comfortable pace going, this can easily be achieved in twenty minutes at a pop during the morning and night, and ten minutes midday. This can also become a source of productive time for you. Try listening to inspirational audiobooks, recording thoughts and ideas on your smartphone or tablet, or socializing with your friends on the telephone.

yoga for the crashed

Yoga therapy can be wonderful. Restorative yoga or Yin yoga classes are your best options. Avoid strenuous yoga, especially "hot" yoga in heated rooms.

reset your sleep pattern

Those who are Crashed usually can get to sleep and stay asleep, but it often does not feel refreshing. Those at this stage often spend too much time in stages of sleep that are less restorative. As the morning cortisol levels start to improve from the ARD and the other tips in this chapter, the quality of sleep often improves noticeably as well. Along with this, it is important to allow your body the time it needs for this sleep to effectively heal your system. This often means eight to ten hours of sleep for the first two to three weeks.

thermal therapy—bathing

Of the many changes that happen when the body's circadian rhythm is disrupted are those that concern how your body controls your temperature. The normal ebb and flow of the body's temperature is especially lacking, and this is behind poor circulation, muscle pain, and poor-quality sleep, which drives the cycle of fatigue further.

Simply taking a few minutes before bed to rest in a lukewarm bathtub can help your body experience better temperature regulation and enjoy more refreshing sleep; the nerves in your skin can help calm the nerves in your brain. For these purposes, the water ideally should not be too cold or too warm. Between 95 and 100 degrees F. is most effective, the closer to body temperature the better. Adding a 2-pound carton of Epsom salts is even more helpful; Epsom salts are magnesium sulfate, which is a mineral often lacking in those whose bodies have put them in survival mode. Epsom salts are absorbed through the skin, so bathing in it can raise your circulating levels of magnesium and improve energy levels, as well as allow for greater muscle relaxation.

wet socks

Improving the circulation leads to better muscular energy, less pain, and fewer fatigue symptoms. Many who are Crashed are aware that muscle pains often disturb their sleep, as do spontaneous movements such as restless leg syndrome. Because our blood is moved about in a closed system, any increase in circulation in one area causes increased circulation elsewhere. Wet socks are an old trick from the days of European hydrotherapy spas that can dramatically improve circulation in just a matter of weeks.

For supplies, you will need two pairs of socks, one long and heavy pair of wool socks and one pair of thin cotton ankle socks. Immediately before going to bed, get the cotton socks wet with room-temperature water and wring them out thoroughly. (If you are prone to chill or intolerant of cold, you can even just wet the half of the socks nearest the toes for your first few treatments.) Put on the cotton socks and place the wool ones on over top of them. The idea is that having water against your skin causes your blood supply to increase to warm the area. Having the wool socks over the top keeps you warm even when your skin is wet, which keeps you from getting chilled. Over the course of the evening, the socks will dry and your feet will get more blood flow, and as stated above, the rest of your muscles will as well.

Most people notice deeper and better-quality sleep with the first session. Try the wet socks nightly; after you level up, you can come back to this trick if you find yourself run down or on the edge of catching a cold.

shedding a little light on light therapy

When you are Crashed, sleep is typically heavy and unrefreshing. This is because there is no big difference between daytime and nighttime cortisol levels. Light therapy can still be helpful, but because the daily cortisol curve is flat, it needs some modifications. Rather than right after waking, start the light therapy ninety minutes afterwards. Rather than thirty minutes, plan for forty-five minutes to help your sleep improve.

On sunny days, spend some time relaxing outdoors. When the sun is not available, do your morning planning or eat your breakfast underneath a light box emitting at least 10,000 lux. Since you are doing this later in the morning, you can also use your light box while working.

adrenal tonics for the crashed

Some supplements have the effect of helping your body tolerate more cortisol or of slowing how fast you eliminate the cortisol. Allowing your adrenals to produce more cortisol is helpful when you are Crashed (but not when you are Stressed or Wired and Tired). Note that many adrenal supplements that include more than 50 mg of basil, or more than 100 mg of pantothenic acid (vitamin B5), can be counterproductive, since they can lower cortisol even further.

morning adrenal tonic: american ginseng

Ginseng is one of the best-known herbal tonics. Many different types, forms, and colors of ginseng exist, each with slightly different effects. In general, ginseng is stimulating and strengthening. These properties are most useful for those who are the very depleted and exhausted.

The root of the American ginseng plant (*Panax quinquefolius*) contains active chemicals called ginsenosides, which have been shown to greatly help with exhaustion and fatigue. Most common effective dosages range from 30 to 100 mg daily.[2] (Those who are Stressed or Wired and Tired may find ginseng to be unpleasantly stimulating.)

morning adrenal tonic: licorice

Licorice (*Glycyrrhiza glabra*) is one of the most useful herbs for underperforming adrenals. It can give many of the benefits of supplemental cortisol with much less risk of side effects and dependency. It can gently raise cortisol levels by helping the body use it longer. For these very reasons, those with higher cortisol levels may experience side effects of fluid retention and blood pressure elevation.

Most standard licorice capsules contain 2 percent glycyrrhizin. At this potency, 30 to 100 mg can be a helpful dose in the morning for adrenal dysfunction.[3] Licorice is also available in tea form and has a taste that people tend to feel strongly about either way. Note that commonly available licorice candies are no longer made from actual licorice and are not useful for adrenal function.

evening adrenal tonic: chamomile

Those who are Crashed may need a little help unwinding. Chamomile tea (*Matricaria recutita*) can be a perfect fit. Chamomile has been shown to lower stress and anxiety without being a sedative and can also improve sleep. It also decreases cramps in the muscles and the intestines.[4]

Chamomile is pleasant tasting and easy to find in supermarkets and even restaurants. This is a hearty plant that grows like a weed in many parts of the country. If you are lucky enough to have some in your backyard, just steep a handful of its flowers in hot water. Chamomile tastes great by itself and it pairs really well with ginger or peppermint.

why not just take cortisol?

The symptoms that go along with being Crashed reflect too little production of cortisol. It seems logical that if a person has too little cortisol, giving cortisol in pill form would be helpful. When someone has Addison's disease and he or she is unable to make cortisol, this is essential. However, the bad side of giving cortisol to someone who does not have Addison's disease is that very quickly the body becomes dependent on it and hence lowers its own output even further.

As the needs of cortisol fluctuate through the day and at different levels of stress, someone who can no longer make his or her own cortisol is in danger of lapsing into acute adrenal crisis, should the individual get sick or have an accident. It is also hard to stop taking cortisol once it has been used for some length of time without experiencing lasting feelings of weakness and dizziness. Darla's story is a clear example of the dangers.

One rainy afternoon, Darla came to see me for the first time. This was memorable partly because the Sonoran desert rarely sees rain but mostly because of Darla's indifference to being wet. As I entered the room and introduced myself, I noticed her papers were wet, her hair was disheveled, and there was water on her face, yet she made no attempts to correct any of this. Before sitting down I knew she was in a state of despondency.

As we spoke, Darla shared that she had been diagnosed with chronic fatigue syndrome several years ago and had gone on long-term disability from her career in social work. She had many health concerns, including her weight and early diabetes, but it became clear that nothing would change with her fatigue in the state that it was. Even though she slept between twelve and sixteen hours a day, she always felt as if she needed more sleep. Every few months she would attempt to walk around the block, only to find herself even more exhausted for the next several days. She had already been on treatment for thyroid disease and was taking cortisol pills. The cortisol gave her a bit more energy for the first few weeks, but caused fluid retention and weight gain.

After evaluating her closely, I explained to her that the cortisol pills were not helping her. Her body was able to make cortisol, but it was not doing so on purpose. Over the next few months I helped her with the Adrenal Reset Diet, supplements including American ginseng and licorice, and light therapy. Within one month Darla was down to sleeping nine to ten hours per day and able to do moderate exercise again. By three months she'd shed 20 pounds and, most important, she had a renewed sense of hope about her future.

➡ clear your mind ... and speed your healing

When you are Crashed, the last thing you need is more demands put on your time, even for things like relaxation and meditation. By doing a three-minute breathing exercise in the morning and passively listening to a guided meditation at night, you can still engage your mind to help speed your recovery.

breathing for energy

Breathing exercises can be helpful in improving overall health and raising vitality. The deep state of fatigue felt at this adrenal level is often accompanied by a sense of coldness. The right type of breathing exercises can radically warm the body and improve energy levels.

Tibetan monks, as far back as the 1700s, used breathing exercises for very practical purposes. Many monasteries were placed far from the bustle of life and often on land parcels that were not already in use for farming, living, or commerce. This often meant remote areas at high elevations, where it was cold. Some monks became so adept at warming their bodies with breathing that they would turn it into a challenge by practicing in rooms just above freezing, covering themselves only with sheets soaked in cold water. Breathing Fire is a modified version of one of their techniques.

> *Step 1:* Sit down with your back straight. If your knees tolerate it, sit kneeling on a cushion on the floor, with your legs folded beneath you. If this is not comfortable, find a straight-backed chair to use. Place something roughly 6 feet in front of you to focus on visually. This can be an image, a piece of jewelry, or any other small thing that is meaningful to you.

> *Step 2:* Holding your gaze on the fixed point, breathe in through your nose and out through your mouth rapidly. While you are breathing, feel your abdomen rising and falling. Imagine you are opening and closing an old-fashioned bellows to blow wind on a fire. Your lower abdomen should be expanding and

contracting like this bellows. Repeat until you have done a few dozen breaths and feel comfortable with the technique.

Step 3: Pick up the pace and count 20 breaths in rapid succession. Imagine with each breath that a loved one is suspended in a cage. All that is keeping him or her safe is a thin rope that is close to being burned through by a candle flame several feet away. Each breath should have the intensity you would use if you were trying to blow out the flame. After the last of the 20 breaths, breathe in as deeply as you can and hold your breath. Challenge yourself to hold your breath as long as reasonably possible.

The first few times you try Breathing Fire, one round may be enough. When you feel ready to try more, you can go straight from the exhalation after holding your breath into another cycle of 20 rapid breaths. If you find yourself dizzy at any point, just breathe gently and move more slowly next time. Practice for three minutes once daily in the morning.

guided imagery: let someone else do the work for you

Today, many great audio programs are available that lead the listener through a series of visualizations to improve health and well-being. These can be used any time of day. A catch-22 for many who are Crashed, however, is that they know stress reduction techniques could help them, but they often lack the mental energy to take on anything new. Guided imagery is a perfect fit because it requires no mental exertion on the part of the participant.

These programs are composed of a guide's voice taking you through a journey of peaceful environments with exercises and questions that elicit security and resilience in the face of future stressors. An excellent visualization called "Guided Visualization to Thrive" can be downloaded from www.adrenalresetdiet.com/resources.

a sample day for crashed

Here is a quick primer on how these techniques can be easily fit in to your day, no matter how low your energy is.

WAKE UP

45 minutes of bright light after being awake for 90 minutes

BREAKFAST

ARD high-protein breakfast

Gentle morning walk for 10 to 20 minutes

American ginseng and licorice

MORNING ROUTINES

Breathing Fire for 3 minutes

MID-MORNING SNACK

Foods from ARD unlimited list

LUNCH

ARD balanced lunch

MID-AFTERNOON SNACK

Healing Juice (page 215)

DINNER

ARD healthy-carb dinner

BEDTIME RITUALS

Guided visualization

Chamomile tea

⟹ leveling up

Since the Crashed level represents the most extreme state of adrenal dysfunction, those who are unassisted can find themselves trapped for a substantial time. Even though this level truly can be a pitfall into which one can continue to plunge, it is also a state that can be moved out of quickly given the right understanding and circumstances. The main focus for recovery is to allow yourself needed rest without expectations or judgments.

Once you begin following the Adrenal Reset Diet and working to minimize your mental, physical, and dietary stressors, this state can completely pass within one to two months. Even if major stressors persist, you can enjoy greater vibrancy and clarity in merely a matter of weeks by using the techniques in this chapter to improve your health.

Stay on top of your progress by retaking the Adrenal Level Quiz (Chapter 5) on the first day of each month. You can get free copies to print at www.adrenalresetdiet.com/resources.

thriving

RECOGNIZING THAT LIFE WITHOUT DIFFICULTY IS SIMPLY NOT possible is a tenet of many of the world's wisdom traditions. "Life is pain," to paraphrase the first of the Buddha's Four Noble Truths. To know what it means to thrive, then, is to recognize this inevitability and to imagine a distinction between pain and suffering. Think of pain as the inevitable traumas we face, great or small. Then think of suffering as our response to those traumas. Thriving should not be thought of as the lack of pain or the lack of suffering but, rather, the art of effective suffering. To thrive is to choose to respond to suffering with resolve and hope rather than despondency.

Another distinction of those who are thriving is that they focus on the stressors they choose rather than on those that are imposed on them. A physical example could be that of experiencing the muscle soreness from a hard workout rather than the back pain from too little movement. In terms of emotional pain, it's the difference between the warm sadness you feel in opening yourself to the pain of a friend in need versus how you feel after the rant of a domineering boss. People who truly thrive realize that life offers many opportunities in which being willing to take on a temporary discomfort means greater happiness later.

In our physical health, thriving is a state in which our adrenal glands respond to stressors, but quickly come back to balance.

Although being educated about managing your health is helpful, this state is not reached by stressing over and micromanaging every small detail. It is important to make educated decisions in those situations where we can choose what to eat and how to care for our bodies. Unfortunately, some of the unhealthiest and unhappiest people I have known were those who knew many rules but had no perspective on which were the most important. Often, when people are in situations in which they cannot meet their ideal standards, they abandon all standards. Even if the salmon is not wild and the spinach is not organic, it is still better than the food from the vending machine. To thrive is to manage your health without being managed by it.

Traveling through Thailand, I was lucky enough to talk in depth with a group of monks of several different ages. The elderly monks, especially, impressed me with their radiant health. Of course, as soon as I felt comfortable doing so, I had to ask about their secrets to wellness: What did they eat? They explained that people in the town gave them each a large bowl of food every day, and they were extremely grateful for it. Later, I saw them receive the food and joyously eat it. Their bowls consisted of every type of Asian food you could imagine: vegetables, rice, seafood, meat, packaged sweets, and sodas. That is varsity-level thriving.

 ## what happens when you're thriving

What is it like when your weight is no longer a struggle? I remember Lorne; he was a patient of mine in his mid-70s. As was routine, my staff recorded his weight and vitals before I came in to see him. When I reviewed these numbers, Lorne was proud to tell me that his weight had changed no more than 3 pounds either way ever since he graduated from high school. My curiosity was piqued. At that particular time, I was gaining weight while cycling twenty hours each week and seeing the failures of the calorie model in the mirror. I thought about the 3,500 calories each pound of weight represented and how Lorne could have been so accurate for all these years. "It's pretty simple," he said. "I eat when I'm hungry and then I quit."

janet's story: an insider's look at "thriving"

One day Janet, a 46-year-old woman, was telling me about her extended visit with in-laws. The moment she said, "Life is still tough sometimes, but I have fun with it now," I knew she was thriving. The year before, she was 17 pounds above her preferred weight and at the Crashed level.

She went on to explain about the visit last month. Her kids already had activities every day and her husband's family ended up staying with them for three weeks. She said, "At first it seemed like it would be too much. I was so busy I wasn't doing my morning walks and I was getting mad. But then I realized that we could have our company help out rather than feel like we had to take care of them. I think they liked the idea, and soon it seemed normal for all to pitch in for dishes and housework. Mind you, we are glad to have our lives back, but we won't be afraid to have them over again soon. Last year, when my adrenals were out of whack, I could not have kept up and I certainly would not have thought of a creative solution like that."

When you are really thriving, that is how it works. If you think about it, the mechanisms that regulate hunger and weight would have to work well for us to survive as a species. If we did not eat enough, we would get malnourished. If we always ate too much, we would run out of food too fast.

When you are thriving you will still get hungry and you still might overdo it, especially when socializing. But when this happens, you will be less hungry for a while and you will spontaneously choose to be more active. It is only when we live our lives in survival mode that our cells so deeply fear famine that the urge to store fat is greater than our body's urge to stay at a stable weight.

too stressed about stress?

By this point it should be clear that stress is not your friend, and it can wreak havoc on your health. Yet hold on a minute—a 2012 study has added a wrinkle to our understanding of how stress affects us. When you really get down to it, your health may have less to do with stress than how you *feel* about your stress.

The data in this study came from a questionnaire about stress taken in 1998 by over 28,000 American adults. The first question was about the level of stress they experienced, and they were also asked how they felt their stress affected their health. Over the next eight years, researchers tracked the public death records of the participants and compared their longevity to their responses in the stress survey. The results showed that stress did predict early death, but to a much greater degree when people *believed* it affected their health. Shockingly, those who were under high stress but did not believe it caused them harm had better health than those with less stress who felt it was more harmful!

We all know how it feels to be stressed. You may feel your heart race, your stomach bind, and your muscles tighten. But how you interpret these feelings may change how they affect you. You can interpret them as signs of irreparable damage being done to your body, or you can interpret them as signs of your body's heroically marshaling of its efforts. Both possibilities are real, and your expectation determines which one will be real for you.

The stress response can improve your focus, aid in your stamina, and help you act decisively. Honor the wisdom of your body for giving you this boost, and you may find the stress won't take the same toll.[1]

your adrenals might be thriving if . . .

The most common cortisol pattern for those who are thriving is levels that are nice and high in the morning and very low during deep sleep.

Typical Cortisol Rhythm: Thriving

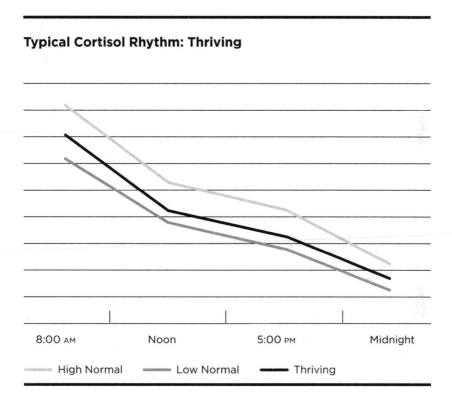

| 8:00 AM | Noon | 5:00 PM | Midnight |

High Normal   Low Normal   Thriving

 the secret to thriving ever more

If you are already thriving, congratulations are in order. It is more likely that you are thriving because you have overcome and managed stressors than because you have had a stress-free life. Continue to pay attention to your exercise, diet, and sleep. When you are thriving, weight loss may still be a goal, or if not, maintaining your weight certainly will be. The Adrenal Reset Diet will easily help with either of these goals. Here are a few more things to consider along the way.

 ## what to add to your ARD eating plan

In terms of your body weight, you will find that it is easier to maintain now than it was in the past. ARD participants have said things like, "It feels like I am immune to fat." "My weight doesn't seem to go up anymore, even during vacations."

Although your body may have reset, weight gain is not impossible. Still, many who follow the ARD are surprised to find that their appetites have completely changed. They do not find themselves as drawn to poor-quality food and they really look forward to eating vegetables. The paradox is, as with so many things in life, that the healthier you are, the easier it is to stay healthy.

Even the inevitable major traumas will have less and less impact over time. Your habits will become so deeply ingrained that they will take on a momentum of their own. You will gain experience in managing unusual situations. After reading this chapter, you will have lots of skills under your belt that allow you to deal with circumstances like travel and changes to your schedule.

Even when you are thriving, it is good to have some clear, written goals regarding your health. Write out your ideal weight, waist circumference, resting heart rate, and any other markers that are important to you. This is also a good time to jot down your other life goals, whether they are a new relationship, career, or skill. Along with this, write down what you plan to do as steps to reach these goals. Share this list with a close friend or your health-care provider and revisit it at least yearly. It is harder to slip up when you know someone else is there to support you.

super you on superfoods

If you are already thriving, how would you like faster weight loss, more energy to chase your dreams, and a stronger immune system to protect you on the go?

Hippocrates said to let your food be your medicine. Vegetables, spices, and fruits are among the best medicines you can find. Here are some of the best foods to have more regularly:

Beets	Dandelion leaves
Cardamom	Dulse
Carob	Ginger
Carrots	Mulberries
Celery	Tomatillos
Daikon	

circadian function reset and repaired

move it right

When you are thriving, exercise becomes play. Rather than forcing yourself to do it, you may feel indulgent or slightly guilty because you are having so much fun with it. You will find yourself wanting to move your body on a regular basis. Have fun with it and consider the following ideas.

cardio

Do all you like and enjoy it. Be aware, though, that if you suddenly increase how much cardio you do, it may push you into survival mode, so build up gradually. Most who are healthy can handle thirty to sixty minutes of aerobic activities four to five days per week. With cardio training, the health benefits increase with the more time you spend—up to about sixty minutes per session.

long slow distance (LSD)

If you are thriving and would like to kick up your fitness even further, you can try LSD a few times each month. No, this is not an illegal drug, although the endorphin rush you get may make you wonder. LSD is gentle, continuous aerobic activity for more than 2½ hours. During this time your glycogen storage lowers and your muscles become better at burning fat. The lasting benefit is that when your muscles burn fat better, your body has less of a need to produce cortisol (which elevates your blood sugar) and you are less apt to have cortisol elevations, even under times of stress. Implement LSD by making it a habit to go for long bike rides or hikes regularly once per weekend. These outings should be undertaken at a leisurely pace and are best done in scenic places with natural beauty. LSD bouts are also a great time to spend quality time with friends and loved ones. We bond and we understand each other best when our bodies are moving.

strength 2.0

Would you look at the set of kidneys on that babe! Sure, lifting weights helps you look good, but did you know that it can also keep your organs healthy? When you are thriving there are no restrictions on exercise, but as a foundation, it is smart to do the types that will help you the most, now and though the years. Without strength training, we gradually lose our lean body mass. This happens to lean mass we see, such as on our thighs and biceps, but it also happens to lean mass we don't see, such as in our kidneys, heart, liver, and bones.

Circuit training is one of the easiest and most effective ways to keep your lean mass healthy. Great upper-body movements include pulling, as in rowing or pull-ups, and pushing, as in overhead presses or push-ups. With your lower body you can do variations on squatting, lunging, and bending at the hip. Choose one exercise for each of the five and do two to five sets of them in sequence. This means doing one set of a squatting exercise, one of pushing, one of lunging, one of pulling, and one of bending. Next, repeat the whole series for the second set. Visit www.adrenalresetdiet.com/resources for ideas on specific exercise options.

be a sport: the beauty of competition

Are you in an exercise rut? Sign up for a 5K. What sports did you love in school? There are adult leagues for nearly every sport and at all levels of abilities. I have adult friends who compete in kickball, soccer, dodge ball, basketball, racquetball, and rowing.

People love games because they have clear goals and set measurements. Think about golf; if the goal were really to get the ball in the hole, you could just walk over and put it in. From kickball to triathlons, more people are doing amateur sports than ever before. Here is a secret: only a small percentage of the "competitors" are really competing. Most are just out to have fun, and some are competing with themselves to beat their personal best.

 # the sweet sleep

When you are thriving, you may find that sleep is one of life's greatest pleasures. The more deeply engaged and awake you are throughout your day, the deeper and more refreshing your sleep will be at night.

try lucid dreaming

Have you ever been in the middle of a dream and realized you were dreaming? If so, you have experienced a lucid dream. *Lucid* means "understandable" or "bright," and both meanings apply to lucid dreams. They are also unique in that you choose what you will dream about. No longer relegated to mysticism, lucid dreaming has become the focus of world-class researchers such as Stephen LaBerge, PhD, of Stanford University.

Developing the basic skills of lucid dreaming not only helps you get to sleep but often provides completely new perspectives on your daily struggles. Over the years, numerous great works of art and inventions have come from those who practice lucid dreaming. Notable persons who used this trick for inspiration include Albert

Einstein, Paul McCartney, Steven King, Edgar Allen Poe, and Rene Descartes.

One of the most effective ways to cultivate the skill of lucid dreaming is as simple as noticing numbers. Make a habit throughout your day to look for numbers in your environment. These can readily be found on calendars, clocks, street signs, elevator buttons, and door labels. When you see a number, make a quick mental note of it, look away, and look back. Of course, in normal life the number will remain unchanged when you glance back at it.

The images and elements within the dream state require a fair amount of our brain's capacity to maintain. If you make looking for numbers a habit in your waking state, you will often find yourself looking for them in the dream state. Typically, our brain does not put forth the effort to maintain consistency in background images like numbers. When you see a number in a dream and look back at it, it will usually be different. This can be used as your cue that you are dreaming.

The second part of lucid dreaming is to make a habit of repeating a word as you fall asleep that represents an understanding you wish to gain from your dreaming mind. In my early days of college, I realized I could never be able to afford to pay for medical school. During a camping trip deep in the woods with only my dog, I used lucid dreaming one night to help figure out a way to make it work. I woke with a sense of clarity about working as a nurse during medical school and looking further for scholarships.

shedding light on light therapy

When you are thriving, light therapy is still useful to maximize your mood and mental productivity. It also helps prevent alterations to your body's rhythms from the number of factors in modern life that can disrupt them. But that's a simple get: all that you need to maintain this is fifteen minutes of bright light exposure during the first hour you are awake. On sunny days, take a nice walk outside or enjoy your breakfast outdoors. On the days when the sun is not an option, bring out your trusty light box.

adrenal tonics for the thriving

Even when you are thriving, who would not want to have even more energy and resiliency? Tonics can be useful to regain energy more quickly after the occasional late night and to keep immunity strong. Some of the best for those who are healthy include reishi and tulsi.

morning adrenal tonic: reishi

Reishi (*Ganoderma lucidum*) is a medicinal mushroom that acts as an adrenal adaptogen. It can help keep your energy levels high without being a stimulant. Since it can keep your immune system strong and protect from pollutants, it is especially helpful when traveling. The most practical way to take reishi is in capsules. Better products contain 10 percent polysaccharides and can be used in doses of 400 to 600 mg twice daily with food.

evening adrenal tonic: tulsi

Tulsi (*Ocimum tenuiflorum*) is a relative of the common culinary herb basil. It has been extensively studied for its abilities to reverse mild depression and prevent cortisol abnormalities. If you find yourself wound up after a full day of exciting challenges, it might be just the thing to help you gently unwind. Regular basil (*Ocimum basilicum*) has many similar properties and can make a reasonable substitute.

If you ever find yourself feeling especially frazzled or close to getting sick, a mega-dose of basil in the form of pesto might be just the tasty ticket. Be sure to check the "Dinners" section of Chapter 10 to find out how to make my favorite pesto.

 clear your mind ... achieve even more

Something funny happens around the time we reach the Thriving level. Many find that their lives are running smoother, with fewer dramas and distractions to manage. When this happens, people start putting more thought into what really matters and what will make them the happiest. Sometimes the answers to these questions are surprising.

hotly pursue happiness

The modern consumer culture teaches us that happiness is easy to find; it is waiting right behind the next purchase. This belief leads to the logical conclusion that the ultimate level of happiness comes from winning the lottery and having the purchasing power this would bring. However, psychologists have found that events that happen to us have shockingly little ability to change our level of happiness, for good or bad.

The most dramatic example I have seen of this was from a study that asked this very question: How much happier do we become if we fall into great fortune? The study also asked the opposite question: How much less happy do we become when we face personal tragedy? To answer these questions, changes in happiness were compared in two groups of people in the months after a major life change. One group won a major lottery. The other group lost the use of their legs from vehicle accidents. For the first few months, the lottery winners were happier than average and the new quadriplegics were less so. This would be expected. But by the time three months had passed, both groups were no more or less happy than they were before the life-changing event. At six months out, this did not change. Lottery winners were no happier than before and new paraplegics were no less.[2]

If the events around us have little power to shape our happiness, then what does?

learning to flow

Mihaly Csikszentmihalyi is a psychologist who made it his life's work to find which circumstances give rise to happiness. He tracked scores of people for decades to learn what created the most positive feelings. He found that we are at our best when we are using our skills in a slightly challenging way to achieve a positive outcome. He called this state "flow." An example could be a manager marshaling her team to perform, a climber summiting a difficult peak, or a parent enjoying the achievement of his child. The types of situations that are most apt to produce flow are those that possess the following three traits:

1. They require use of a skill that took substantial time to acquire.

2. They have an appropriate level of complexity. Activities that are much too difficult are not conducive to flow, nor are those that are far too easy. Ideally the tasks increase in complexity to meet the increased level of ability.

3. They serve some useful purpose. The most beneficial activities for us are those that are also beneficial for others.

To the extent we can, it is advisable to adapt our careers and direct our pastimes toward activities that keep us in a state of flow. This may be achieved by learning new skills on a regular basis. Try picking up a few new hobbies each year; these can include physical ones like kayaking, mountain biking, or Pilates. Mental activities are also great; some include learning the basics of a foreign language or even how to do basic web publishing. Csikszentmihalyi showed that these experiences occurred most often at work or during structured play.

embrace the power of community

How important is community to us? Think about this: How can you punish someone who is already in prison? Solitary confinement. Humans are social animals; having no contact with others can be among the most traumatic experiences. Not only does isolation cause early death, but it also has been shown to lead to obesity.[3]

Even when we are simply in the presence of others, our level of community can be thought of on a continuum. It is entirely possible to be isolated even when not confined. Those who have frequent meaningful interactions with loved ones and extended family members consistently show better health and longevity.

In 1966, researchers noticed that the men in Roseto, a small Pennsylvanian town, seemed immune to heart disease even though they had poor diets and high rates of smoking. It was also noticed that Roseto had a highly connected community and had crime rates much lower than average. People knew each other well and helped each other as needed. When their analysis was completed, Roseto's researchers attributed exceptional health to their high level of community.[4]

What can the rest of us model from that? Interacting with people is every bit as medicinal as broccoli and push-ups. Little things like going to movies or cultural events can lower stress and keep your body thriving. Staying connected with friends and family can take some small effort, but that effort is clearly worthwhile.

helper's high

If you really want to get ripped, try working in a soup kitchen. Seriously, one of the most effective ways to get healthy has nothing to do with traditional weight-loss advice. You have learned that lowering your total level of stress helps you stay lean. What is the most efficient ways to lower your stress? Focus on someone else's.

Dr. Allan Luks coined the term "Helper's High" to refer to the positive changes that come from assisting others. When you help someone, you get an initial feeling of euphoria, followed by a lasting sense of calmness. Clearly that sounds more like thriving than like surviving. Dr. Luks has monitored thousands of people, and he has shown that those who regularly assist others are ten times more likely to be healthy.[5]

Dr. Luks findings were confirmed in a study that tracked 10,317 Wisconsin residents from 1957 to 2008. Those who volunteered on a regular basis were over 60 percent less likely to die than people at the same age who did not. Along with lower mortality, volunteering was shown offer benefits: "happiness, life satisfaction, self-esteem, mastery, depression, and physical health."[6]

Here are a few insights from digging deep into the data from the Wisconsin study: (1) helping several organizations is less effective than focusing on one or two; and (2) you can get all the health benefits from volunteering with as few as 40 hours per year.

Only 40 hours per year. Imagine that—45 minutes per week can help you lose weight, lower depression, and extend your life. The only side effect is that you are making the world a better place!

What are the most practical ways to do this? Along with traditional volunteering, there is mentoring and working toward social change. Skills that we take for granted, like driving, reading, and doing household tasks, could completely change the day for someone in need. Mentoring is great for those who have a specific professional skill. Help out someone new to your industry or encourage those considering it. Participating in social change is a great option if you find yourself stressed about the state of society. Find the one issue that is the most important to you and partner with others who feel the same. Environmental concerns, faith-based programs, or policy-changing coordinated activities are all great ways to spend some time.

a sample day for the thriving

When you are thriving, health comes easily but still does benefit from some attention. Use tonics like reishi and tulsi on a regular basis, engage in recreational exercise, and stay laser-focused on your mission of making the world a better place!

WAKE UP

Thirty minutes of bright light within the first hour

BREAKFAST

ARD high-protein breakfast

Unlimited exercise

MORNING ROUTINES

How can you go into "flow"?

Reishi tea

LUNCH

ARD balanced lunch

ANYTIME VACATION

How can you deepen your sense of community?

DINNER

ARD healthy-carb dinner

BEDTIME RITUALS

Journal: Who can you help tomorrow?

Tulsi tea

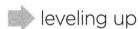 leveling up

When you are thriving, what is there to hold you back? Processed food has been dealt with by carb cycling; physical stressors are less traumatic with better circadian rhythms; and the pressures of life are more manageable with the extra clarity you have gained. The biggest barrier facing those who are thriving is to sink into passivity. Feeling bad about your weight or your health can be a powerful motivator. Once things start to improve, some of that motivation can be lost and it can be easy to let the occasional lapse grow into the resumption of all the old habits.

Passivity can best be remedied by experiencing greater levels of contribution in life. We learned from studies on volunteers that anything you do to help others can also help you. Find ways to share your journey with others. This can be helpful even if you are at different stages along life's path.

- Enlist a walking buddy for your daily walk.

- Bring healthy dishes and recipes to the office.

- Secretly replace your co-workers candy stash with raw almonds (sometimes new members of my team experience this firsthand).

- When people ask how you lost weight, share what truly worked for you. Visit www.adrenalresetdiet.com/resources for a printable one-page synopsis of the book.

Now that you understand the Adrenal Reset Diet, weight loss is no longer a matter of low-calorie snacks and leg warmers; it is a matter of developing flow in your life, building a community, and contributing to others.

Remember: our bodies and lives are constantly changing, whether we intend them to or not. By understanding this and orchestrating the changes with your higher goals, anything is possible. Never give up on yourself, and you'll continue to thrive.

adrenal reset menus and recipes

THE FOLLOWING ARE SOME RECIPES MY FAMILY AND I LOVE TO eat on a regular basis. They are carefully chosen to use the best ingredients, be easy to prepare, and most important, taste great.

Once you understand the basic concepts of the Adrenal Reset Diet, it is not hard to use any of your current favorite recipes with these guidelines. Paleo or low-carb recipes just need the right amount of rice or beans added at the right time. Other recipes may just need to chuck a small amount of carbs and perhaps add some protein to make them work.

make it easy on yourself: plan to succeed

One of the most common barriers is the perceived lack of time. Did you know that the average adult now spends five hours per day on television and social media? If we reduce these daily distractions by even one-third, there is plenty of time to prepare healthy food. Here is another secret: with a little planning, you can make healthy meals in less time than it takes for trips to get fast food.

the art of shopping

Think of your shopping in two categories: trips to maintain your staples and other trips to pick up perishables. Many staples can be purchased in bulk or online, saving both time and money. Fruits and vegetables can be purchased from farmers' markets or from delivery services. Most communities have services that will bring seasonal, organic produce to your home (or nearby) each week. You can even let them know what types of produce you like. Our family has done this for years. The kids love going to the porch each Friday morning to see what we received for the week. Grocery delivery is another great option. Many stores allow online ordering and delivery within a window of a few hours, with minimal delivery charges. We have automated deliveries set up for each week.

pantry staples

WHOLE GRAINS

Black rice

Brown rice

Buckwheat

Quinoa

Wild rice

BEANS AND LEGUMES, DRIED OR CANNED

Adzuki beans

Black beans

Black-eyed peas

Butter beans

Cannellini beans

Garbanzo beans (chickpeas)

Great northern beans

Lentils

Lima beans

Navy beans

Peas

Pinto beans

Red beans

COOKING OILS

Coconut

Macadamia

Olive

Rice bran

NUTS AND SEEDS, RAW AND UNSALTED

Almonds

Chia seeds

Flax seeds

Macadamia nuts

Pistachios

Pumpkin seeds

Sesame seeds

Sunflower seeds

PROTEIN SOURCES (AVOID OILS AND FLAVORINGS; IDEALLY CHOOSE LOW-SALT VARIETIES)

Canned chicken

Canned clams

Canned oysters

Canned salmon

Canned sardines

Protein powder, animal or vegetable based

SEASONINGS

Better than Bouillon brand condensed stock

Capers

Cumin, seeds and ground

Fennel seeds

Garlic

Ginger, fresh and ground

Mustard

Pepper

Red pepper flakes

Sea salt

Vanilla extract (pure)

SWEETENERS

Lo-han (monkfruit)

Stevia

Xylitol

perishables

VEGETABLES

Artichokes

Arugula

Asparagus

Bell peppers, especially red and yellow

Bok choy and baby bok choy

Broccoli

Cabbage

Carrots

Cauliflower

Celery

Chinese (napa) cabbage

Cucumbers

Eggplant

Fennel

Garlic

Green leafy vegetables

Jicama

Kale

Leeks

Lettuce (red, green, or romaine)

Mushrooms

Okra

Onions

Parsnips

Potatoes

Scallions

Shallots

Spinach

Squash (summer and winter)

Sweet potatoes

Swiss chard

Tomatoes

Watercress

FRUITS

Apples

Bananas

Berries

Cherries

Figs (fresh)

Kiwifruits

Lemons

Limes

Pomegranates

POULTRY AND MEATS

Buffalo

Chicken (dark and white meat)

Game (venison)

Grass-fed beef

Pork

Turkey (dark and white meat)

SEAFOOD (BEST OPTIONS BASED ON MERCURY, PCB CONTENT, AND SUSTAINABILITY)

Abalone

Arctic char

Bass

Catfish (farmed)

Clams

Cod (Atlantic)

Crab

Halibut

Lobster

Mussels (farmed)

Oysters

Sablefish (Alaskan)

Salmon (Alaskan wild-caught)

Scallops (wild)

 hacking your kitchen

Most parts of a meal can be purchased pre-cooked. When you are busy, meal preparation becomes less about cooking and more about assembly. Pre-cooked poultry and prepped vegetables are available in nearly every supermarket. Organic brown rice and quinoa are available pre-cooked in nonperishable containers. All types of beans are available canned, ideally organic and low sodium. Grains can be purchased both dried and batch cooked.

Rice cookers make it easy to prepare grains. All you do is add one part dried grains and two parts liquid and press a button. The cooker steams the batch until it is perfectly done and keeps it warm until you are ready to eat. Most even have timers so you can have a batch of rice or quinoa ready to go when you get home from work.

Fruits and vegetables can also be prepped in advance or purchased ready to use. Choose one day per week to cook your staples and prep your produce. In an hour or so you can be ready for the whole week and have some quality time to spare.

What type of cookware is best? I prefer well-seasoned cast iron for sautéing and stir-frying, and heavy stainless-steel saucepans for simmering. Cast-iron pans can work for simmering but sauces that are tomato or citrus based can leach extra iron. Aluminum and nonstick pans both leach endocrine-disrupting chemicals into the food. Porcelain-lined saucepans can contain lead residues and stainless-steel and glass cookware make food stick.

sample menus

You already know that you can keep the ARD as simple as is needed for your lifestyle. If the thought of cooking scares you, know that all of the recipes below are simple, fast, and scrumptious. The menu is just a sampler, and you may not have the inclination or desire to cook every meal for a week in this way. No worries. As long as you remember the ARD carb-cycling rules, you can't go wrong. And don't forget your unlimited vegetable list!

DAY OF THE WEEK	BREAKFAST	LUNCH	DINNER
Monday	California Dreaming Breakfast Soup, page 211	Southwest Chipotle Salad, page 229	Stir-fried Beef, page 239
Tuesday	Tart Smoothie, page 209	Turmeric Chicken Lettuce Wraps, page 226	Seasoned Rice and Veggies, page 232
Wednesday	Lean and Green Smoothie, page 208	Mushroom Muffins, page 230	Carrot Chicken Soup, page 237
Thursday	Lower-Carb Muesli, page 214	Seared Cod with Chilled Potatoes, page 224	Sweet Pea Chicken Soup, page 234
Friday	Reset Parfait, page 210	Salmon Waldorf Salad, page 228	Ground Turkey Casserole, page 233
Saturday	Breakfast Chili, page 213	Spinach Bean Soup with Shrimp, page 231	Poached Salmon in Lemongrass, page 235
Sunday	Cherry Vanilla Shake, page 207	Shrimp with White Bean Salad, page 227	Curried Garbanzo Stew, page 238

shaking off the pounds— a quickstart guide to basic shakes

I learned when I was 12 that the easiest high-quality breakfast was a protein shake. Good breakfasts are just so hard to miss otherwise. People are rushing out the door in the morning, with little time to cook and eat. Mothers often prepare food for everyone else and have that much less time for a proper meal for themselves. By starting the shake habit, you can have a healthy breakfast made and eaten in a matter of minutes, with no prepping and minimal cleanup.

What to Put in Your Shake

Protein

Nonallergenic protein powders are best to prevent food-intolerance reactions. Look for ones that are derived from clean animal protein or peas and are free of other additives, flavorings, or fillers. It should provide 24 to 35 grams of protein per serving and have no added sugar. Examples can be found at www.adrenalresetdiet.com/resources.

Fiber

Seeds and fiber supplements are great additions to your smoothie and they will help keep you feeling full for hours. The best seeds to use are flax, chia, or hemp. Each of these brings a ton of benefits; they are rich in fibers, protein, and essential minerals, and they have unique properties that help your body's detoxification processes. It works well to have several types of seeds on hand and to rotate between them.

Fiber supplements are another option. If the rest of your diet is good and you are using plenty of seeds and vegetables, they are not essential and so not necessary. If used, these should contain a blend of soluble and insoluble fiber, and be free of herbal laxatives, flavorings, or colors. Please note that anytime you change your fiber intake it is good to raise your water intake by 1 cup. Some people notice gas and bloating the first few days when adding more fiber to their diets; this does stop with time as it reflects the bowel flora changing in a good way. Start with a few teaspoons of seeds and ½ teaspoon of any fiber supplement for the first two weeks. From there you can gently work up to 2 tablespoons seeds and a full serving of any fiber supplement you choose.

Greens

Green veggies are superstars at helping weight loss. Your morning shake is a great place to work in another serving or two. Most mild-tasting greens can go right in a shake and have no effect on its flavor. Greens can call for some prep time and they can have a short shelf life. The easy way to work around these concerns is to use frozen greens. Frozen spinach is easy to find and keep. Just toss ½ cup into the bottom of your blender before adding the other ingredients; this lets it mix in thoroughly. Frozen kale also works well.

Other good greens to use include red and green leaf lettuces, romaine, Swiss chard, and cabbage. Many stores have pre-washed and prepped versions of these, making them very convenient. Owing to their stronger taste, some greens aren't as nice in shakes. Think about whether collards, mustard greens, arugula, and turnip greens are too strong for your palate and either don't use them or use them only in tiny amounts.

Liquid

Some type of liquid is needed for the ingredients to blend properly. Water works fine for this, but some people like the taste and texture of a milk substitute. Unsweetened flax milk is my favorite option; it is tasty, nonallergenic, sugar free, and has a great creamy texture. It has one-half to one-third the calories of dairy milk or other milk substitutes, and is even a good source of those hard-to-find omega-3 fats.

If your store does not have flax milk yet, unsweetened coconut milk is the next best option. Please note that this is not the canned condensed coconut milk for cooking but, rather, the coconut beverage in soft packs found in the dairy case or on boxed on shelves in the baking section, along with the soy and almond milks. This is also not the same as coconut water, often found in cans or soft packs. Be aware, though, that unsweetened coconut milk is dense in calories and is best used in quantities of ½ to 1 cup, at the most.

Tasty Things

Along with the essentials mentioned above, consider adding in a few items to round out your shake's flavor and nutrients. Berries are the best option for this purpose. They contain great flavor, additional fiber, and tons of antioxidants.

How can you tell which foods are the healthiest? Easy; it is the ones that stain your clothes the most when they spill. It is true: some of the healthiest chemicals found in plants are the pigments that give them color. In terms of high amounts of flavor and low amounts of sugar, all the berries work well. Blackberries, raspberries, and strawberries have half the fructose of blueberries.

Berries are the fruits of plants grown above ground, and they are not peeled before eating, so it's worth getting organic versions for your health. In terms of fiber content, blackberries and raspberries are superstars, giving up to 8 grams of fiber per cup.

Pre-made Shakes

There are days where every second of time saved can be a treasure. There are also times during dieting when having consistent, pre-measured ingredients speeds progress immensely. For these reasons, pre-made shake mixtures can be useful.

What to Look For

The best mixtures will be consistent with the science behind the Adrenal Reset Diet. They will prevent insulin spikes, allow for healthy cortisol rhythms, and encourage your body to use its own fat for fuel rather than create new fat. So they will also be free of sugars, artificial sweeteners, stimulants, MSG, and other ingredients that can alter cortisol levels. Look for 24 to 35 grams of complete protein, ideally from nonreactive (nontoxic protein) sources. One of my favorites is a cool new option called hydrobeef. It is a powdered version of clean, lean animal protein with a neutral flavor. It is free of fat and contaminants and mixes easily. The other good option is vegetable protein powders from bean sources. For the fibers, a mixture of soluble, insoluble, and resistant fiber is important, while folic acid is best avoided since a high percentage of the population has adverse reactions to it. (Product reviews and information about the mixture used in the ARD study can be found at www.adrenalresetdiet .com/resources.)

Making Your Shakes

You'll need a blender. The higher-end blenders can be nice if you use really hard ingredients like carrots or kale stems, but the Adrenal Reset Shake basic recipe works fine with any blender.

Juicers won't work well for making shakes. They do make

smooth beverages, but in doing so they take out the fiber and many of the minerals. They also cause the liquid to be metabolized more like sugar, which can disrupt the insulin and cortisol balance. If that is not reason enough, juicers take upwards of 15 minutes to properly disassemble and clean after each use.

Once you have your ingredients in mind, just drop them into a blender jar and turn the machine to its highest setting. Rarely is more than 1 minute needed to get it to a good consistency.

Here is a cool trick to clean your blender. After pouring out your smoothie, fill the blender jar about half way with hot water, and add a few drops of dish soap and a few shakes of salt. Blend at medium speed, rinse a couple times, and voilà—it's immaculate and ready for tomorrow!

breakfasts

 shake recipes

If you get bored with the shakes in the Quickstart Guide, here are a few more ideas. Unripe bananas are called for in the following recipes; these are ones that have some green left on the skin and have no brown spots. At this stage, the bananas have a completely different effect on cortisol than when they are ripe. To keep bananas from ripening, peel them in advance and keep in the freezer.

chocolate almond shake

If you have not tried cacao nibs yet, this is a great time to start! If you like a little crunch in your shake, just add them at the very end of the blending.

Serves 2
Prep time: 2 minutes

- 2 servings animal- or vegetable-based protein powder
- 1 cup unsweetened coconut beverage
- 2 tablespoons organic almond butter
- 1 tablespoon organic cacao nibs
- ¼ cup instant oatmeal
- Stevia, to taste

Place all the ingredients in a blender and blend for 2 minutes, adding water, if needed, for desired consistency. Serve immediately and enjoy.

Vegan modifications: none needed

tropical green tea smoothie

Green tea is rich in catechins, which improve metabolism and break down free radicals. Matcha green tea powder is the type used in Japanese tea ceremonies. If you are very caffeine sensitive, try using 1 cup brewed decaf green tea instead. I just put a bag of decaf green tea in a small water container the night before and refrigerate it. By morning it is perfect for this.

Serves 2
Prep time: 2 minutes

   2 servings animal- or vegetable-based protein powder
   1 cup unsweetened coconut beverage
   1 teaspoon matcha green tea powder
   ½ unripe medium banana
   1 tablespoon ground flax seeds
   ½ cup frozen spinach leaves
   Stevia, to taste

Place all the ingredients in a blender and blend for 2 minutes. Add water, if needed, for desired consistency. Serve immediately and enjoy.

Vegan modifications: none needed

cherry vanilla shake

Cherries are wonderful foods if you are prone to gout or arthritis. They also reduce oxidized cholesterol. Frozen dark sweet cherries work really well in this. On occasion, you can also serve ½ cup of the cherries in a bowl as your carb servings in the evening. They are great just as they are.

Serves 2
Prep time: 2 minutes

> 2 servings animal- or vegetable-based protein powder
> 1 cup unsweetened coconut beverage
> ¼ cup frozen or fresh pitted cherries
> 1 teaspoon pure vanilla extract
> ¼ cup instant oatmeal
> Stevia, to taste (optional)

Place all the ingredients in a blender and blend for about 2 minutes, adding water, as needed, for desired consistency. Serve immediately.

Vegan modifications: none needed

lean and green smoothie

Avocado works great in shakes and smoothies. This is an ARD version of your standard tomato cocktail, but with a twist.

Serves 2
Prep time: 2 minutes

> 2 servings animal- or vegetable-based protein powder
> 1 cup cold water
> 1 ripe medium avocado, pitted and peeled
> 2 Roma (plum) tomatoes
> 1 cup fresh or frozen spinach
> ½ unripe medium banana

Place all the ingredients in a blender, adding additional water as needed for desired texture. Blend for about 2 minutes. Serve immediately.

Vegan modifications: none needed

tart smoothie

We love making these with fresh lemons from our yard. Sour tastes can help jump-start digestion in the morning.

Serves 2
Prep time: 2 minutes

  2 servings animal- or vegetable-based protein powder
  1 cup unsweetened coconut beverage
  Juice of 1 lemon or 2 limes
  1 unripe medium banana
  2 tablespoons chia seeds
  Stevia, to taste (optional)

Place all the ingredients in a blender, adding water as needed. Blend about 2 minutes, then serve immediately.

Vegan modifications: none needed

reset parfait

When you are in a rush but want something more solid than a shake, parfaits are a perfect answer. These work best when made the night before and refrigerated

Serves 2
Prep time: 3 minutes

> 2 cups unsweetened coconut beverage
> 2 servings vanilla-flavored animal- or vegetable-based protein powder
> ½ cup oat bran
> ½ cup flax seeds
> 1 cup diced banana (about 1 medium; to prevent insulin spike use unripe bananas)
> ⅛ teaspoon almond extract
> Liquid stevia or powdered xylitol, to taste (optional)

Place all the ingredients except the almond extract and sweetener in a 1-quart mixing bowl. Mix well. Stir in the almond extract, and add the sweetener, if using. Serve immediately or refrigerate for up to 24 hours.

Vegan modifications: none needed

california dreaming breakfast soup

This is one of our favorite and easiest breakfasts. Make a large batch, throw it in the refrigerator, and you have a few days' worth of breakfasts ready to go. Besides, soups always taste even better after they have had some time for flavors to mingle. They work great along with or instead of a smoothie on busy days. Any leftover vegetables can be added, or you can add quinoa or brown rice for a great complete meal later in the day.

Serves 4
Prep time: 3 minutes
Cook time: 2 minutes

> **2 ripe medium avocados, pitted and peeled**
> **1 quart organic chicken or vegetable broth**
> **½ teaspoon ground turmeric**
> **2 chicken breasts, cooked and diced**
> **½ teaspoon ground ginger**

Place the avocado pulp, broth, and turmeric in a blender and blend until smooth. Pour into a 2-quart saucepan. Add the diced chicken and the ginger to the pan and gently heat until warm. Serve warm or refrigerate for up to 72 hours.

Vegan modifications: use vegetable broth and substitute 1 package tempeh or 1 cup cannellini beans for the chicken

chocolate pudding

This is an amazing dish that even the fussiest of eaters will love. Please note that this works best when made the night before, so its flavors combine as it refrigerates; also, the chia seeds won't "pop" without sitting at least a few hours.

Serves 4
Prep time: 3 minutes, plus overnight

> 2 cups unsweetened coconut milk
>
> 1 slightly ripe banana, diced
>
> ¼ cup unsweetened cocoa powder (or carob powder if you are Crashed or caffeine sensitive)
>
> 1 serving vanilla-flavored animal- or vegetable-based protein powder
>
> ½ cup chia seeds
>
> ½ cup sunflower seeds
>
> 1 teaspoon pure vanilla extract
>
> Liquid stevia or powdered xylitol, to taste (optional)

Mix all the ingredients except the sweetener in a 1-quart mixing bowl. Add the stevia or xylitol, if desired. Cover and place in the refrigerator overnight, then serve chilled.

Vegan modifications: no changes needed, it's already there!

breakfast chili

Chili for breakfast? Try it and see how much your metabolism skyrockets! With spices, resistant fiber, veggies, and quality protein, this chili will power your day like no other. It's my favorite breakfast; typically I make a large batch on Sunday evening and am set with breakfasts for the coming week.

Serves 4
Prep time: 3 minutes
Cook time: 13 minutes

- 1 pound 95% lean ground beef or turkey
- 2 teaspoons macadamia or rice bran oil
- 1 cup mild salsa (lower-salt and sugar-free versions; or try salsa verde for an exotic taste)
- 1 tablespoon chili powder
- 1 cup canned black beans, rinsed
- 2 cups arugula or other lettuce
- Optional veggies: onions, mushrooms, cabbage, celery, green chilis, etc.
- Optional garnishes: diced onion, cilantro, parsley, lime wedges

Brown the meat in the oil in a 2-quart saucepan over medium heat, about 3 minutes. Add the salsa, chili powder, beans, and greens. Gently heat until the greens are wilted, about 5 minutes. Add the veggies and cook until tender, about 5 minutes. Garnish with onion and herbs, if using. Serve with lime wedges.

Vegan modifications: omit the ground meat; serve the chili with a protein shake

lower-carb muesli

Maximilian Bircher-Benner was a Swiss physician who developed muesli around the turn of the last century as a breakfast for patients in his hospital. It was inspired by a mixture he and his wife used while hiking in the Swiss Alps. Oats are used in this low-carb version. In their raw state, oats are high enough in resistant starch to not cause significant insulin production.

Serves 4
Prep time: 3 minutes

- ½ cup organic gluten-free old-fashioned rolled oats
- 1 cup shredded unsweetened coconut flakes
- ½ cup freeze-dried or frozen unsweetened blueberries
- 1 teaspoon pure vanilla extract
- Liquid stevia, to taste (optional)

Mix the oats, coconut, and blueberries in a 1-quart mixing bowl. Stir in the vanilla. Add stevia, if using. Enjoy!

Variation: Serve with 1 cup flax milk or ½ cup unsweetened coconut beverage.

juices

Vegetables and fruits are the best snacks, but they can take more time to prepare and eat than you may have available. Juices are the perfect remedy for this time-starved situation. In just a few minutes, you can make an incredible snack to enjoy right away and have some to share with a loved one, or for yourself later in the day.

Juices can be made in a blender or an extraction juicer. Both can be effective tools that make getting healthy amounts of produce much easier. Extraction juicers make a juice with a very smooth consistency; blenders make a juice with more fiber and require less cleanup time. If you already have a unit that you like, stick with it. If you do not, consider one of the several great brands of high-powered blenders on the market, such as Blendtec, Vitamix, or Ninja.

When using a blender, add 1 cup water and 1 cup ice cubes to each blending. Add more water as needed to help the mixture blend. When using a juicer, be sure to add the pulp back into the juice or use it in soups.

Many of these juice ingredients can be purchased already cleaned, cut, and prepped. If you take advantage of this option and use a blender, the whole process can take no more than two minutes, start to finish. If some recipes have ingredients that are new to you, seek them out and try them. Alternatively, the recipes still taste and work great if you have to leave out something you can't find or dislike. Additionally, look at the Resources at the back of the book for ideas on availability of these exact formulas in juice bars in your area.

WHAT DO ALL THE JUICE INGREDIENTS DO?

Avocado	Rich in fiber, essential fats, magnesium, and vitamin B5 (which regulates adrenal function)
Banana (unripe)	High in resistant fiber, which lowers appetite, stabilizes blood sugar, and helps weight loss
Basil	Lowers production of cortisol, improves immune function, kills viruses
Beet	Directly lowers cortisol, aids in detoxification through betaine, heals blood vessels
Broccoli sprouts	Richest known dietary source for detoxifying; contains cancer-protecting compounds known as sulfurophanes
Cacao (cocoa)	Rich in magnesium, can lower cortisol, high in antioxidants
Carrot	Rich in phenols that aid in detoxification, regulates circadian rhythms, and heals skin and connective tissues
Cayenne	Boosts immunity, improves metabolism, helps circulation, reduces inflammation
Celery	Speeds elimination of cortisol, lowers blood pressure; rich in phthalides that relax muscles
Chamomile	Gentle sedative; relaxes muscles, improves depth of sleep
Chia	High in omega-3 fats, which balance adrenal function; rich in fiber and calcium

Cilantro	Effective at preventing absorption of toxins from the intestinal tract; rich source of chlorophyll
Coconut	Boosts mental function, improves tissue repair, improves cortisol metabolism
Cucumber	Reduces inflammation; high in molybdenum, which improves pituitary regulation of adrenal glands
Dandelion leaf	Reduces fluid retention, speeds the liver's breakdown of fatty acids
Ginger	Helps digestion, reduces inflammation, improves immune function
Grapefruit	Rich in enzyme that slows cortisol breakdown and helps prevent insulin resistance
Green apple	High in phenols that aid in detoxification; rich in fiber
Green tea	High in catechins, which speed metabolism and help energy and weight loss
Hemp	High in omega-3 fats; high in GLA, which is a natural relaxant
Kale	Most powerful dietary antioxidant per USDA ranking, rich in chlorophyll
Lemon	High in vitamin C, which improves adrenal function; natural antibiotic; reduces inflammation
Maca	Safe energy tonic

Mint	Improves digestion, improves memory loss; gentle sedative
Orange	Rich in vitamin C, which lowers cortisol
Parsley	High in vitamin K, which helps bone growth and adrenal function; protective against cancer
Pomegranate	Rich in anthocyanins; speeds cortisol elimination; lowers inflammation
Red cabbage	Contains anthocyanins and dithiolethiones, which can regulate the elimination of stress hormones
Spinach	More nutrients per calorie than any other food; rich in magnesium, which regulates adrenal function
Spirulina	Rich source of B vitamins, chlorophyll, antioxidants, and fiber
Tomato	Rich in lycopene, an antioxidant that improves blood sugar metabolism and helps weight loss
Turmeric	Lowers free-radical damage, lowers inflammation, helps liver function; antiviral

juice recipes

Each juice recipe makes two servings, or approximately 16 fluid ounces (2 cups, or 1 pint). Each recipe has the same steps:

(1) Place all the ingredients in a high-powered blender and add 1 cup water and 1 cup ice cubes.

(2) Blend for at least 2 minutes. Serve.

thriving juice mix

2 medium beets, peeled and quartered

1 handful baby carrots (about 1 cup) or 2–3 large carrots, cut into smaller pieces

3 celery stalks

½ inch slice fresh ginger, or ¼ teaspoon ground ginger

2 Roma (plum) tomatoes

1 cup frozen chopped spinach, or 2 cups fresh spinach leaves

stressed juice mix

2 medium beets, peeled and quartered

3 celery stalks

½ inch slice of fresh ginger, or ¼ teaspoon ground ginger

1 cup frozen chopped kale, or 2 cups fresh kale leaves

1 medium orange, peeled, seeded, and quartered

½ cup pomegranate seeds, or ¼ cup pomegranate juice

wired and tired juice mix

2–3 fresh basil leaves, or ½ teaspoon dried basil

1 handful baby carrots (about 1 cup), or 2–3 large carrots, cut
   into smaller pieces

2 tablespoons chia seeds

1 large cucumber, peeled and cut into chunks

1 medium green apple, cored and quartered

1 cup frozen chopped spinach, or 2 cups fresh spinach leaves

crashed juice mix

½ medium avocado, peeled, pitted, and cut into chunks

1 slightly unripe banana

½ grapefruit, peeled and quartered

1 tablespoon powdered maca root

½ bunch fresh parsley, stems trimmed

2 cups chopped red cabbage

½ inch sliced fresh turmeric, or ¼ teaspoon ground turmeric

more healing juices

Along with the specific recipes to reset your adrenals, here are some tasty recipes for meeting other health goals and to provide some variety.

Each juice recipe makes two servings, or approximately 16 fluid ounces (2 cups, or 1 pint). Each recipe has the same steps:

(1) Place all the ingredients in a high-powered blender and add 1 cup water and 1 cup ice cubes.

(2) Blend for at least 2 minutes. Serve.

gentle detox juice mix

- 2 medium beets, peeled and quartered
- ½ cup broccoli sprouts
- ½ bunch fresh cilantro, stems trimmed
- 1 medium green apple, quartered and cored
- ½ cup frozen chopped kale, or 1 cup fresh kale leaves, stem removed
- ¼ lemon, sliced and seeded
- ½ inch sliced fresh turmeric, or ¼ teaspoon ground turmeric

smooth skin juice mix

½ medium avocado, peeled, pitted, and cut into chunks

1 handful baby carrots (about 1 cup), or 2–3 large carrots,
     cut into smaller pieces

3 celery stalks

½ cup unsweetened fresh coconut

1 large cucumber, peeled and cut into chunks

4–6 fresh mint leaves, or ½ teaspoon dried

immune boost juice mix

4–6 fresh basil leaves, or ½ teaspoon dried basil

2 cups fresh or frozen blueberries

1 handful baby carrots (about 1 cup), or 2–3 large carrots,
     cut into smaller pieces

¼ cup dried goji berries

¼ lemon, sliced and seeded

lean juice mix

1 pinch of cayenne pepper

1 cucumber, peeled and cut into chunks

1 cup fresh dandelion leaves

½ inch slice fresh ginger, or ¼ teaspoon ground ginger

½ grapefruit, peeled and quartered

1 medium green apple, quartered and cored

2 Roma (plum) tomatoes

energy lift juice mix

- 1 slightly unripe banana, peeled
- 1 tablespoon unsweetened cocoa powder or cacao nibs
- ½ cup unsweetened fresh coconut
- 1 cup green tea
- 1 tablespoon ground maca root
- 1 cup frozen chopped spinach, or 2 cups fresh spinach leaves
- ½ teaspoon Spirulina

calm juice mix

- 2 medium beets, peeled and quartered
- 3 celery stalks
- 2 tablespoons hemp seeds
- 4 fresh mint leaves, or ½ teaspoon dried mint
- ½ cup pomegranate seeds, or ¼ cup pomegranate juice

lunches

seared cod with chilled potatoes

If carbs have gotten a bad rap, potatoes have taken the brunt of it. Ironically, potatoes can make the unhealthiest food (potato chips) and also be one of the healthiest (chilled boiled potatoes). Potatoes have resistant starch, but it is destroyed when cooked at high temperatures, such as when baking or frying. Boiling preserves much of that starch, and when the boiled potatoes are refrigerated they form even more starch in a process called retrograde resistant starch formation. Green beans do this to some degree also.

Serves 4
Prep time: 5 minutes
Cook time: 10 minutes

- 1 teaspoon macadamia nut oil
- 1 pound wild-caught Atlantic cod fillet
- 1 pound baby potatoes, boiled 20 minutes, then refrigerated overnight
- 1 pound green beans, boiled 10 minutes, then refrigerated overnight
- ¼ cup diced red onion
- 1 tablespoon soy-free vegan mayonnaise

Heat the oil in a large sauté pan on medium-high heat. Sear the cod fillet for 3 to 5 minutes on each side, until flaky. Allow the cod to cool slightly, then cut it into small pieces. Dice the potatoes and beans, and mix with the onion in a large bowl. Add the cod and then spoon in the mayonnaise and stir gently. Serve immediately or pack the salad into a container, refrigerate, and serve later.

Vegan modifications: none available

salmon teriyaki with asparagus

If you try this dish you'll learn that teriyaki can be great even without all the extra sugar that most versions have.

Serves 4
Prep time: 5 minutes, plus 30 minutes marinating
Cook time: 10 minutes

- **1 pound wild-caught Atlantic salmon fillet**
- **2 tablespoons mirin**
- **1 teaspoon toasted sesame oil**
- **¼ cup tamari or wheat-free soy sauce**
- **1 pound asparagus, ends removed, spears cut into 2-inch sections**

Cut the salmon into four portions. In a large bowl, make a marinade by mixing the mirin, sesame oil, and soy sauce. Add the salmon pieces and the asparagus and refrigerate for at least 30 minutes or up to overnight.

Preheat the oven to broil. Remove the salmon and asparagus from the marinade and place on a cooking sheet. Broil for 4 minutes on each side or until the asparagus is slightly softened and salmon starts to flake. Serve warm. If bringing the salmon to work as a lunch, pack it in a container with ½ cup steamed brown rice. Save the rest in the fridge for family or other meals.

Vegan modifications: none available

turmeric chicken lettuce wraps

Turmeric is an amazing plant, and in cooking we enjoy its
rhizome, or swollen root. If you can find fresh turmeric, it is
worth the effort; most Asian supermarkets stock the rhizomes.
It looks just like fresh ginger, but when you cut into it, the color
is that of a carrot. It is also sold commonly in powdered form.

Serves 2
Prep time: 3 minutes, plus several hours to meld flavors

- 1 pound chicken tenderloins, cooked
- 2 tablespoons soy-free vegan mayonnaise
- 1 teaspoon ground turmeric, or 1 tablespoon grated fresh
  turmeric
- 1 pinch of freshly ground black pepper
- 1 teaspoon lime juice
- 1 cup canned cannellini beans, rinsed
- 8 large romaine lettuce leaves

Place all the ingredients except the lettuce leaves in a large
serving bowl and mix thoroughly. Refrigerate for several hours
or overnight. Divide evenly into servings, and spoon the mixture
onto the leaves. Form wraps and serve.

Vegan modifications: omit the chicken; add 1 scoop vegetable-
based protein powder, and increase the beans to 2 cups

shrimp and white bean salad

Shrimp is a great protein option. Look for wild-caught bay shrimp, rock shrimp, Gulf pink shrimp, or U.S. farmed shrimp.

Serves 2
Prep time: 5 minutes, plus chilling time

    4 cups lettuce, washed and torn (escarole, endive, or romaine)
    8 ounces cooked shrimp, deveined and peeled
    1 sprig fresh cilantro, chopped
    1 cup canned white beans, rinsed
    1 red bell pepper, diced
    ¼ cup diced red onion
    1 large celery stalk, diced
    1 tablespoon extra-virgin olive oil
    3 tablespoons red wine vinegar
    1 teaspoon ground cumin

Place all the ingredients in a 2-quart mixing bowl and toss gently and thoroughly. Cover and refrigerate until ready to serve.

Vegan modifications: omit the shrimp; increase the beans to 2 cups

salmon waldorf salad

The original Waldorf salad includes apples, walnuts, and celery. This version is quick to prepare and makes a complete meal. In fact, it's perfect for lunch. The recipe will make enough for you and another adult or child. You can also keep it all for yourself and eat half for lunch the following day. If you do plan to save some of the salad, add the dressing just before you are ready to eat it.

Serves 2
Prep time: 10 minutes

SALAD

- 6 cups lettuce, washed and torn (escarole, endive, or romaine)
- 6 ounces canned wild salmon packed in water, drained
- 1 Granny Smith apple, quartered, cored, and diced
- 6 walnut halves
- 2 celery stalks, diced
- ½ cup canned garbanzo beans (chickpeas), rinsed

DRESSING

- 2 tablespoons soy-free vegan mayonnaise
- 2 teaspoon dried tarragon

Place all the salad ingredients in a 2-quart mixing bowl; combine the dressing ingredients and add to the salad; toss thoroughly. Serve immediately or refrigerate until ready to eat.

Vegan modifications: omit the salmon; increase the garbanzo beans to 1½ cups

southwest chipotle salad

Chipotles are smoked jalapeño peppers, which have a unique flavor; they are available canned but also as a powder. Do not despair if you are not a fan of spicy foods. Small amounts of chipotle seasoning give more flavor than heat. Make a few days' worth of this salad in advance. Just remember to add the dressing right before serving.

Serves 4
Prep time: 5 minutes, plus optional chilling time

SALAD

- **8 cups greens, washed and torn (romaine, spinach, or shredded cabbage)**
- **2 cooked chicken breast halves, diced**
- **½ cup finely sliced red onion**
- **2 cups broccoli florets**
- **1 cup cherry tomatoes**
- **2 cups canned black beans, rinsed**

DRESSING

- **½ cup unsweetened coconut beverage**
- **1 ripe medium avocado, peeled and pitted**
- **⅓ cup fresh lemon juice**
- **1 garlic clove, crushed**
- **¼–½ teaspoon chipotle seasoning, or a few shakes of Tabasco sauce**

Place all the salad ingredients in a 2-quart mixing bowl. In a separate bowl, whisk together the dressing ingredients. Pour the dressing over the greens and toss thoroughly. Cover and refrigerate for 30 minutes before serving, if possible.

Vegan modifications: omit the chicken

mushroom muffins

This is a one-dish meal with great flavor, tons of fiber, good-quality protein, and lots of antioxidants. You can whip up one or two batches of these in no time and have a portable and tasty lunch ready to go.

Makes 12 muffins; 2–3 muffins = 1 serving
Prep time: 10 minutes
Cook time: 25 minutes

4 teaspoons macadamia or rice bran oil
2 cups sliced button mushrooms
1 red bell pepper, diced
1 small red onion, diced
2 garlic cloves, minced
½ teaspoon sea salt
½ teaspoon freshly ground black pepper
½ teaspoon chili powder
½ teaspoon ground turmeric
1 cup cooked or canned green lentils, rinsed
1 cup diced cooked chicken breast
½ cup garbanzo bean (chickpea) flour

Preheat the oven to 350°F. Add 1 teaspoon of the oil to a heavy-bottomed pan and sauté the mushrooms, red pepper, and onion over low heat until softened, about 3 minutes. Add the garlic and other seasonings and stir. Add the lentils and chicken, and mix thoroughly. Add the flour and blend but do not overmix.

Coat the cups of a muffin tin with remaining 1 tablespoon oil, then spoon in the mixture, filling the cups nearly to the top. Bake for 20 to 25 minutes or until firm. Serve warm, or refrigerate and then reheat when ready to eat.

Vegan modifications: omit the chicken, and substitute 1 scoop unflavored vegetable-based protein powder; blend thoroughly before baking

spinach bean soup with shrimp

Here is another great lunch dish that can be made in the morning before you go to work (it's that easy!). Bring a batch for your co-workers; they will be amazed at your culinary skills. You don't have to tell them it only took 20 minutes. Note that this recipe uses canned coconut milk, which is not the same thing as the coconut milk in soft packs that I suggested using with your shakes.

Serves 4
Prep time: 5 minutes
Cook time: 15 minutes

   1 teaspoon macadamia or rice bran oil
   1 small red onion, diced
   1 pound cooked shrimp, deveined and peeled
   1 can (1½ cups) coconut milk
   1½ cups canned black beans, rinsed
   ½ cup chopped raw cashews
   1 garlic clove, minced
   ½ teaspoon freshly ground black pepper
   ½ teaspoon sea salt
   1 teaspoon chili powder
   1 pinch cayenne pepper
   6 cups fresh spinach leaves

Heat the oil in a 2-quart heavy-bottomed saucepan and sauté the onion until softened, 1 to 2 minutes. Add the shrimp and cook for 1 minute. Then add all the remaining ingredients except the spinach, and simmer over low heat for 10 minutes. Stir in the spinach and cook until wilted, about 1 minute more. Serve warm or refrigerate for up to 24 hours (for best flavor) and reheat when ready to eat.

Vegan modifications: omit the shrimp; add 1 serving vegetable-based protein powder

dinners—the evening feast

seasoned rice and veggies

Even if you are not vegetarian or a vegan, it is fine to have an occasional vegetarian dinner. Make sure it is high in fiber and that it has some healthy carbohydrates, and stick with a single serving.

Serves 4
Prep time: 10 minutes
Cook time: 40 minutes

- 1 cup brown rice
- 2 cups vegetable broth
- 2 teaspoons toasted sesame oil
- 1 cup quartered button mushrooms
- ½ cup diced white onion
- ½ cup sliced zucchini
- ½ cup sliced red pepper
- 1 teaspoon grated fresh ginger
- 1 tablespoon miso paste
- ⅓ cup pine nuts
- ¼ cup diced fresh cilantro (optional)

Rinse the rice, then add it and the broth to a 2-quart saucepan. Cover and simmer on low heat for 30 to 40 minutes. Meanwhile, add the sesame oil to a heavy-bottomed saucepan and sauté the mushrooms, onion, zucchini, red pepper, and ginger until the vegetables start to soften, about 3 minutes. Mix in the miso paste and pine nuts, cook 1 minute more, then fold the rice in with the vegetable mixture. Sprinkle with cilantro, if desired. Serve warm.

Vegan modifications: none needed

ground turkey casserole

If your evenings are really tight, consider preparing this in the morning and putting it in to bake when you get home. Cook the quinoa ahead of time or buy it pre-cooked. Serve this as a stand-alone dish or with a mixed green salad. This recipe has a handwritten "A+" in our family cookbook. Being from the Midwest, I'm naturally a casserole connoisseur.

Serves 4
Prep time: 5 minutes
Cook time: 25–30 minutes

- 1–2 teaspoons macadamia or rice bran oil
- 8 ounces lean ground turkey
- 1 cup diced sweet onion
- 1 cup canned navy beans, rinsed
- 1 cup unsweetened coconut beverage
- ½ teaspoon sea salt
- ½ teaspoon freshly ground black pepper
- 1 teaspoon ground turmeric
- 1 teaspoon ground coriander
- 1½ cups sliced or pre-shredded carrots
- 1½ cups chopped asparagus (1-inch pieces)
- 2 cups shredded green cabbage
- 1 cup vegetable broth (or 1 cup water plus 2 teaspoons Better than Bouillon)
- 2 cups cooked quinoa

Preheat the oven to 350°F. Place the oil in a large skillet and sauté the turkey and onion over low heat until the turkey is browned, about 3 minutes. In a blender, combine the beans, half the coconut beverage, and the spices, spinning until smooth. Combine the turkey-onion mixture, blender contents, and remaining ingredients in a large casserole dish. Bake, uncovered, for 25 to 30 minutes. Serve warm.

Vegan modifications: omit the turkey, and substitute 1 serving unflavored vegetable-based protein powder

sweet pea chicken soup

Here is a fresh twist on split pea soup. There's no mushiness and there's a much nicer color green.

Serves 4
Prep time: 5 minutes
Cook time: 10 minutes

1½ cups diced onions
1 tablespoon macadamia oil
2 garlic cloves, minced
½ teaspoon freshly ground black pepper
2 teaspoons ground cumin
3 cups vegetable broth (or 1 tablespoon Better than Bouillon
    vegetable base with 3 cups water)
3¼ cups frozen peas
2 cups diced cauliflower
¼ cup diced raw cashews
1 teaspoon ground cinnamon
1 teaspoon paprika
½ teaspoon salt
1½ pounds skinless and boneless chicken, cooked and diced

In a large stockpot, sauté the onions in the oil over medium heat until soft, about 3 minutes. Add the garlic, pepper, cumin, and 2 tablespoons broth and sauté an additional minute. Add the peas and cook until bright green. Let cool slightly, then puree the pea mixture in your blender.

Place this pea base back in the stockpot, add remaining ingredients, and simmer an additional 3 to 5 minutes. Serve warm, or refrigerate until ready to use. It will keep for up to 72 hours.

Vegan modifications: use thawed tempeh in place of the chicken

poached salmon in lemongrass

A family favorite! Choose a wild-caught Atlantic salmon fillet that is fresh and firm. If you cannot find fresh lemongrass, dried can work, too. We also use essential oil of lemongrass for dishes like this; you can easily find it online, and it has a shelf life of years. If you do use it, however, be sparing as a little goes a long way. Most dishes need only a tiny drop or two.

Serves 4
Prep time: 5 minutes
Cook time: 10 minutes

    2 quarts water
    4 green tea bags
    2 tablespoons minced fresh lemongrass, or 4 tablespoons dried
        lemongrass
    1 teaspoon sea salt
    1 pound fresh salmon fillet, in 4 pieces
    2 cups diced broccoli

Place the water, tea bags, and lemongrass in a large saucepan. Bring to a low boil, remove from heat, and let sit for 5 minutes. Remove the tea bags and lemongrass and discard them. Add the salmon pieces and simmer gently for 5 minutes, or until the outer flesh starts to flake. Add the broccoli and simmer for an additional 3 minutes. Serve with steamed brown rice (recipe follows).

Vegan modifications: none available

steamed brown rice or quinoa

Healthy grains are great staples to always have cooked and ready to go in the refrigerator. Chicken or vegetable broth can be used. My family loves Better than Bouillon brand stock paste, since it has only clean ingredients and is more versatile than broth. This can be done on a stovetop, but rice cookers make it so much easier!

Serves 8
Prep time: 2 minutes
Cook time: 45 minutes

> **2 cups long-grain organic brown rice or organic quinoa**
> **2 teaspoon Better than Bouillon vegetable base or chicken**
>   **flavor, or 2 cups vegetable stock**
> **2 cups water**

Rinse the rice. Add the rice, bouillon base, and water to a 2-quart stockpot or rice cooker. Simmer lightly, covered, over low heat until all the water is absorbed, roughly 45 minutes. Serve warm or refrigerate for up to 72 hours.

Vegan modifications: none needed

carrot chicken soup

This recipe provides a unique blend of flavors and it's easy to pre-cook. Many supermarkets now stock organic pre-shredded carrots, which makes cooking this even easier.

Serves 4
Prep time: 5 minutes
Cook time: 20 minutes

2 tablespoons macadamia oil
1½ cups chopped white onions
1 tablespoon grated fresh ginger
1 teaspoon ground cinnamon
½ teaspoon chili powder
4 cups shredded carrots
¾ cup fresh orange juice
2 cups unsweetened coconut beverage
2 cups chicken or vegetable broth
1 teaspoon salt
½ teaspoon freshly ground black pepper
1½ cups diced cooked chicken breast

Place the oil in a large soup pot and then add the onions. Sauté until softened, about 3 minutes, then add the ginger, cinnamon, and chili powder. Sauté an additional minute. Add the carrots, orange juice, coconut beverage, and broth and bring to a simmer. Simmer for 10 minutes, until the carrots are soft. Add the salt and pepper and the chicken, and simmer an additional 5 minutes. Serve warm or refrigerate for up to 72 hours.

Vegan modifications: omit the chicken (use 1 pound thawed tempeh instead, if desired)

curried garbanzo stew

Curry is a blend of spices, usually built around turmeric. There is a compound found in turmeric called curcumin that can do more for your health than almost anything else. It helps control blood sugar, lowers inflammation, may reduce the risk of cancer, and supports the immune system. In fact, extracts of curcumin work as well for pain and inflammation as do medications like ibuprofen—and without the side effects.

Serves 4
Prep time: 5 minutes
Cook time: 15 minutes

> 2 teaspoons macadamia or rice bran oil
>
> 1 teaspoon mustard seeds
>
> 2 teaspoons cumin seeds
>
> 2 cups chopped green cabbage
>
> 1 cup diced white onion
>
> 1 teaspoon grated fresh ginger
>
> ½ fresh jalapeño pepper, seeded and minced (wash hands carefully after handling)
>
> 1 cup pureed tomatoes
>
> 1 teaspoon dried turmeric
>
> 1½ cup canned garbanzo beans (chickpeas), rinsed
>
> 1½ cups cooked brown basmati rice, kept warm
>
> ½ cup chopped fresh cilantro (optional)

Heat the oil in a large skillet and add the mustard and cumin seeds over high heat until they pop, about 2 minutes. Add the cabbage, onion, ginger, and jalapeño, and cook until all have softened, 2 to 3 minutes more. Add the tomatoes, turmeric, and garbanzo beans. Simmer for 5 to 10 minutes. Serve hot over the rice, sprinkled with cilantro, if desired.

Vegan modifications: none needed

stir-fried beef

Choose lean cuts of grass-fed beef, such as sirloin or skirt steak. There are some nutrients that beef is really rich in; zinc, taurine, conjugated linolenic acid, carnitine, vitamin B12, and iron are just a few. The grass-fed varieties also offer some omega-3 fats, as are found in fish. This recipe goes well with steamed brown rice (page 236), making it a complete meal.

Serves 4
Prep time: 2 minutes
Cook time: 10 minutes

> **1 teaspoon toasted sesame oil**
> **1 pound boneless beef steak, sliced for stir-fry**
> **2 pounds bok choy, sliced, stems and leafy parts separated**
> **2 garlic cloves, minced**
> **2 pinches freshly ground black pepper**
> **1 pinch sea salt**

Heat the sesame oil in a large skillet and sauté the steak over medium heat until browned, about 3 minutes.

Add the bok choy stems and garlic and sauté about 1 minute more. Add bok choy leaves and sauté an additional 5 minutes. Season with pepper and salt. Serve hot over rice.

Vegan modifications: Use 1 pound thawed tempeh instead of the beef

basil pesto

This sauce/seasoning works great as a topping for pasta or chicken.

Serves 4
Prep time: 10 minutes

  2 cups organic fresh basil leaves, loosely packed (roughly
    4 ounces)
  1 garlic clove, cut in half with green kernel removed
  ¼ cup extra-virgin olive oil, or more as needed
  Juice of 1 lemon
  ½ cup pine nuts, raw and shelled

Place the basil, garlic, oil and lemon juice in a blender. Blend, stirring and adding additional olive oil, if necessary for consistency, until a smooth green paste is formed. Add pine nuts and blend just enough to break them into large pieces. Use immediately or store in the freezer; it keeps well.

Vegan modifications: none needed

just the faqs

Any questions? Start right here.

which foods should i avoid?

public enemy #1: fructose

Fructose will not always be labeled as sugar in ingredient lists. Ingredients are listed in descending order of quantity, and food manufacturers often use several types of sugar, so sugar does not appear as high up on the list as if the types were combined. Some names for various sugars to look out for include:

Agave, agave nectar

Barley malt

Beet sugar

Brown rice syrup

Brown sugar

Cane juice, cane sugar

Caramel

Carob syrup

Castor sugar

Coconut sugar

Confectioner's sugar

Corn syrup, corn syrup
 solids

Date sugar

Dextran

Dextrose

Diastatic malt

Ethyl maltol

Evaporated cane juice

Fructose

Fruit juice, fruit juice concentrate

Galactose

Glucose, glucose solids, glucose polymers

Granulated sugar

Grape sugar

High fructose corn syrup

Honey

Icing sugar

Invert sugar

Jaggary

Lactose

Maltodextrin

Maltose

Malt syrup

Maple syrup

Molasses

Muscovado sugar

Organic sugar

Pearl sugar

Raw sugar

Refiner's syrup

Rice syrup

Sorbitol

Sorghum syrup

Sucrose

Sucunat

Sugar in the raw

Superfine sugar

Treacle

Turbinado sugar

public enemy #2: toxic proteins

Some proteins trigger the survival mode. It is important to identify and avoid them to lose weight. How much does this matter? In 2009, a group of twenty-seven people were studied who had failed to lose weight on low-calorie diets. Each participant was tested for food reactions, and they were instructed to avoid their reactive foods. Foods that commonly caused these reactions were wheat, eggs, and dairy. Within twelve weeks, members of the group went from an average weight of 200.6 pounds to an average of 163 pounds. The average amount of weight lost was 37 pounds, with a reduction in body fat from an average of 37 percent to 27 percent.[1]

Toxic proteins include the following sources of wheat, dairy, and eggs:

WHEAT

Biscuits	Pancakes
Bread	Pasta
Breakfast cereals	Pizza crust
Cakes	Pretzels
Couscous	Rolls
Croissants	Scones
Danishes	Waffles
Muffins	

DAIRY

Butter	Ice cream
Buttermilk	Kefir
Cheese	Milk
Cottage cheese	Sour cream
Cream-based salad dressings	Whey protein
Cream-based soups	Yogurt

EGGS

Albumin	Egg solids
Baked foods	Egg whites
Batters	Egg yolks
Egg noodles	French toast
Egg protein	Macaroons

Marshmallows

Mayonnaise

Pancakes

Waffles

Wheat noodles

how many times per day should i eat?

If you feel fine with three meals a day, do not push yourself to eat more often. Despite the claims, there is no magic way that eating more frequently makes you lose weight. It is true that each time you eat, a percentage of the calories is lost to the process of digestion. Compare this to the idea that buying on sale is the same as saving money. Even if something is 30 percent off, you are still spending money.

Having said that, if you feel better with light snacks between meals, it is a great time to work in a few extra servings of vegetables. Keep some combination of baby carrots, celery, cauliflower, or broccoli florets on hand. Look at the unlimited food lists for more ideas, or go to the juices section in Chapter 10.

which should be my biggest meal?

The food you eat in the morning helps regulate your day's metabolism and blood sugar levels, but it is not burned for fuel that day. Since it takes eight to sixteen hours to process food, most of each day's fuel comes from the evening before. Our ancestral pattern was to hunt and wander throughout the day, with occasional light grazing. The main meal was often in the evening around a communal campfire.

Later on, when agriculture was the prime source of food, the main meal was typically in the evening, after work was completed. We carry this over to today, with the evening being the most logical time to socialize and have the main meal.

The Adrenal Reset Diet makes the evening meal the day's largest. This schedule reduces hunger, increases weight loss, improves depth of sleep, and lowers the stress response.

should i have a cheat meal?

There is strong evidence that the body's metabolism can deal with the occasional feast. When you are at your target weight, having such a cheat meal once a week is fine, but until then, alternating weeks is best. It is important to plan this cheat meal in advance and have it in the evening; this way your muscles will get more of the food than your fat will. Many people like their cheat meal on Sunday evenings, and they will eat a lighter than normal breakfast and lunch beforehand.

Whenever you find yourself craving a particular food during the week, do not tell yourself "no." Tell yourself "later." Make a note on your schedule of what it was you wanted and promise yourself that you can have it when the cheat meal comes around. Please note that the cheat meal is a meal, not a "cheat evening." Gather together anything and everything you think you want to eat, and sit down with it. Once you are full and you get up from the chair, the cheat meal is over.

what if i am vegetarian or vegan?

If you have chosen to avoid eating foods of animal origin, for ethical or spiritual reasons, do not despair. The Adrenal Reset Diet can still work just fine for you. Vegetarian and vegan options are available for all elements of the diet.

If you avoid animal protein for health reasons, kudos to you for putting serious thought into it and for being brave enough to break common habits. When done right, plant-based diets can have a lot going for them. If there is one thing that the nutrition world agrees on, it's that our diets need more fresh produce, more fiber, less sugar, and fewer cured and processed meats.

As you likely know, the hard part in a vegetarian diet is getting *optimal* protein. Please note that I did not say *adequate* protein. The difference between adequate and optimal can be compared to other nutrients, like vitamin C. If you do not get adequate amounts of vitamin C, you will develop scurvy; this can be prevented with as little as 5 to 7 mg of vitamin C per day. Yet all nutritionists agree that, scurvy aside, 75 to 120 mg is an optimal intake. The same concept applies to protein. To lose fat and get lean, it takes getting 20 to 30 percent of your calories from protein.[2]

Please know that you dietary needs may change over time. It is healthy to think of your diet as an ongoing conversation; those who thrive are the people who respect the feedback they receive from their bodies and honor its changing needs.

does "gluten free" mean it is okay?

Over the last few thousand years, the wheat plant has been cultivated extensively and has developed proteins that can be problematic. Many people now have celiac disease and milder versions of gluten intolerance. Thankfully, there is more awareness of these problems and more gluten-free foods available. However, just because something is labeled "gluten free" does not guarantee that it is good for you.

When an intact whole grain, like a kernel of brown rice, is made into flour, that flour will get digested more quickly like sugar. Scores of unprocessed foods are naturally gluten free; they include fish, poultry, seafood, meat, nuts, seeds, fruits, vegetables, eggs, rice, buckwheat, quinoa, and beans. Alternatively, gluten-free replacements for bread, cereals, and snacks might be made with poor-quality ingredients. If you suspect you have a gluten intolerance, get tested and find out. (Suggestions for obtaining accurate testing can be found at www.adrenalresetdiet.com/resources.) It is possible to be reactive to foods even if they do not make you feel worse right after eating them—that is, there may be a delayed reaction. Whether or not you have a problem with gluten, it is best to focus your diet on simple, unprocessed foods.

what is my problem with beans?

As much as it is sometimes a joke, gas from eating beans can be a problem for many people. Thankfully, a recent large study proved

that this is a passing problem, no pun intended. In the study, participants were given ½ cup of beans of various types daily. At the beginning, 35 percent of the group felt that they were having more gas
than normal. By the second week, this was down to 19 percent. By
the fifth week, only 5 percent still had extra gas, and by the eighth
week it was down to 3 percent.

Some of the biggest bean offenders are pinto beans and navy
beans. If you are new to beans, it may be best to leave these out
of your diet for the first few months. Black-eyed peas are a good
"gateway bean" because they cause the least problems for new users.
If beans have been a problem for you, start with 2 tablespoons of
black-eyed peas daily for two weeks. From there you can add in different types and different amounts without risking social problems.[3]

Apart from gas, some people are concerned about eating beans
because of a chemical called phytic acid, also called inositol hexaki-
sphosphate, or IP6. Beans do contain it, but so do many other foods.
In fact, nuts and seeds have the highest amounts of phytic acid. It is
true that it slows absorption of some minerals, but it also has been
shown to protect against many types of cancer. Naturally occurring
amounts of phytic acid in the context of a healthy diet are not worrisome, and may even have some health benefits.

which sweeteners are okay?

Clearly, sugar is unhealthy. But are artificial sweeteners any better?
Evidence is growing that artificially sweetened foods can also lead
to weight gain. So which sweetener is best to use? The main considerations are whether it is toxic, how much fructose it has, and how
it affects the blood sugar.

Cane sugar (granulated, superfine, confectioner's), brown sugar
(cane sugar coated with molasses), molasses, raw sugar, and turbinado sugar do badly on all counts. Sucralose (Splenda) and aspar-
tame (Nutrasweet) can be toxic and can disrupt the blood sugar.
Agave nectar, honey, and coconut sugar are high in fructose, which
is hard on the liver and causes the most weight gain.

Stevia and monkfruit (also known as lo-han) are plant extracts that have a sweet taste but no calories. Both have been thoroughly studied and shown to be safe. They even have some antioxidants and help blood sugar. The one drawback is that they can taste bitter. Your best option is to try a few different brands of pure stevia and monkfruit, and see which one tastes the best to you.

the reset redux—
the diet in a nutshell

When our bodies shift into survival mode, we gain weight. Survival mode also disrupts sleep and raises our reactions to stress (see table that follows). Processed foods, pollutants, and the pressures of life trigger this physiologic pattern. Typical weight-loss efforts, like eating less and exercising more, only make the problem worse. By cycling your carbohydrates, repairing your circadian rhythms, and raising your mental clarity, you can make yourself resistant to the survival mode, lose weight, and thrive!

PROBLEMS	PROCESSED FOOD	POLLUTANTS	PRESSURES OF LIFE
Details	Fructose Toxic proteins	Environmental Light	Relationships Work Finances
Consequences	Adrenal Fat Switch gets set to survival mode. Hunger increases, energy decreases, and food is stored as fat.		

CURES	CARBOHYDRATE CYCLING	CIRCADIAN REPAIR	MENTAL CLARITY
How	Low Carb in AM High Carb in PM	Improved sleep Daily detox Tonics	Brain exercises Daily habits
Results	Adrenal Fat Switch resets to Thriving mode. Hunger lowers, energy increases, and food is burned for fuel.		

start today diet plan

breakfast = protein shake

Blend the following ingredients with ice and water:

- 1 serving animal- or vegetable-based protein powder
- ½ cup raspberries
- 2 tablespoons chia seeds
- ¼ cup canned navy beans

lunch = mixed salad

- 1 palm-size piece salmon or chicken, unlimited greens, and low-starch veggies; avoid corn, potatoes, and sweet potatoes
- ½ cup canned kidney or garbanzo beans (chickpeas)
- 1 tablespoon olive oil and vinegar, as needed

dinner = stir-fry

- 3–4 ounces lean beef or chicken, unlimited veggies
- 1 cup cooked brown rice or quinoa
- Tamari soy sauce, ginger, garlic, 1 teaspoon toasted sesame oil

snacks = veggies, any type, any amount, anytime

See page 80 for list of veggies

resources

CUSTOM ARD SUPPLEMENTS

www.drchristianson.com/supplements

JUICE BARS WITH ARD JUICE FORMULAS

Grabba Green: see www.grabbagreen.com for locations

HOME TESTING OPTIONS

Food allergies: www.drchristianson.com/testing

Hair cortisol: www.drchristianson.com/testing

Salivary cortisol: www.drchristianson.com/testing

HOME THYROID QUIZ

www.thethyroidquiz.com

LIGHT THERAPY MACHINES

Day-Light Sky 10,000 LUX Bright Light Therapy Lamp

Carex Health Brands Day-Light Classic 10,000 LUX SAD Lamp

SOUND LIGHT MACHINES

MindPlace Proteus USB Light & Sound Meditation Mind Machine

DAVID Delight—Audio Visual Entrainment

acknowledgments

I'd like to thank the following people for making this book possible. Thanks to my parents, Glen and Vivian Christianson, for giving me a love of learning and confidence in my own ideas. Thanks to my wife, Kirin, for believing in me, and to my children, Celestina and Ryan, for bringing me joy each day. To my other father, Dr. David Frawley, for inspiring me to write. Thanks to the incredible team at Integrative Health with whom I am lucky to spend my days: Sharon Anderson, Dr. Lauren Beardsley, Tipton Billington, Melissa Bogardus, Celia Cacciotti, Easton Lathion, Jamie Kurtz, Miranda Baigneault, Dr. Linda Khoshaba, Michele Lambert, Kim Lopata, Dr. Saman Rezaie, Dr. Tonyelle Russell, Mary Cinalli, Jennifer Stadig, Dr. Adrienne Stewart, and Ashley Ross. Special thanks to JJ Virgin for showing me a greater vision of what was possible. Thanks to my world-class literary team, Scott Hoffman and Heather Jackson, with whom I am honored to work. Thanks to my favorite external brain, Sara Gottfried, MD, who helped shape these ideas. Thanks to Drs. Michael Murray, ND, Paul Mittman, ND, and Michael Cronin, ND, for their roles in defining and expanding our profession. Final thanks to my lifelong hero, the late Dr. Carl Sagan, for his unparalleled passion and eloquence in sharing the grandest ideas.

notes

INTRODUCTION

1. Doetsch R. 1978. "Benjamin Marten and his 'New Theory of Consumptions.'" *Microbiological Reviews* 42(3):521–28.

CHAPTER 1

1. Ogden CL, Fryar CD, Carroll MD, and Flegal KM. 2004. "Mean body weight, height, and body mass index, United States 1960–2002." Advance data from vital and health statistics, no. 347 (Hyattsville, MD: National Center for Health Statistics).

2. Murray CJL, and Lopez AD. 2013. "Measuring the Global Burden of Disease." *New England Journal of Medicine* 369(5):448–57. doi: 10.1056/NEJMra1201534.

3. Mann T, Tomiyama J, Westling E, Lew AM, Samuels B, and Chatman J. 2007. "Medicare's search for effective obesity treatments: Diets are not the answer." *American Psychologist* 62(3):220–33.

4. Young BE, Johnson SL, and Krebs NF. 2012. "Biological determinants linking infant weight gain and child obesity: current knowledge and future directions." *Advances in Nutrition* 3(5):675–86. doi: 10.3945/an.112.002238.

5. Klimentidis YC, Beasley TM, Lin HY, Murati G, Glass GE, Guyton M, Newton W, Jorgensen M, Heymsfield SB, Kemnitz J, Fairbanks L, and Allison DB. "Canaries in the coal mine: a cross-species analysis of the plurality of obesity epidemics." *Proceedings of the Royal Society: Biological Sciences* 278(1712):1626–32. doi: 10.1098/rspb.2010.1890.

6. Goldstein RE, Wasserman DH, McGuinness OP, Lacy DB, Cherrington AD, and Abumrad NN. 1993. "Effects of chronic elevation in

plasma cortisol on hepatic carbohydrate metabolism." *American Journal of Physiology* 264(1 Pt 1):E119–27.

7. Wei Y, Wang D, Topczewski F, and Pagliassotti MJ. 2007. "Fructose-mediated stress signaling in the liver: implications for hepatic insulin resistance." *Journal of Nutritional Biochemistry* 18(1):1–9.

8. Legeza B, Balázs Z, and Odermatt A. 2014. "Fructose promotes the differentiation of 3T3-L1 adipocytes and accelerates lipid metabolism." *FEBS Letters* 588(3):490–6. doi: 10.1016/j.febslet.2013.12.014.

9. Gabriely I, Hawkins M, Vilcu C, Rossetti L, and Shamoon H. 2002. "Fructose amplifies counterregulatory responses to hypoglycemia in humans." *Diabetes* 51(4):893–900.

10. Lomer MC, Parkes GC, and Sanderson JD. 2008. "Review article: lactose intolerance in clinical practice—myths and realities." *Alimentary Pharmacology and Therapeutics* 27(2):93–103.

11. Eswaran S, Goel A, and Chey WD. 2013. "What role does wheat play in the symptoms of irritable bowel syndrome?" *Journal of Gastroenterology and Hepatology* (NY) 9(2):85–91.

12. González-Cervera J, Angueira T, Rodriguez-Domínguez B, Arias A, Yagüe-Compadre JL, and Lucendo AJ. 2012. "Successful food elimination therapy in adult eosinophilic esophagitis: not all patients are the same." *Journal of Clinical Gastroenterology* 46(10):855–8. doi: 10.1097/MCG.0b013e3182432259.

13. Wilders-Truschnig M, Mangge H, Lieners C, Gruber H, Mayer C, and März W. 2008. "IgG antibodies against food antigens are correlated with inflammation and intima media thickness in obese juveniles." *Experimental and Clinical Endocrinology and Diabetes* 116(4):241–45.

14. Costa-Pinto FA, and Basso AS. 2012. "Neural and behavioral correlates of food allergy." *Chemical Immunology and Allergy* 98:222–39. doi: 10.1159/000336525.

15. Schreier HM, and Wright RJ. 2013. "Stress and food allergy: mechanistic considerations." *Annals of Allergy, Asthma, and Immunology.* 2014 Feb;112(2):179–181.e2. doi: 10.1016/j.anai.2013.08.002.

16. Wang J, Sun B, Hou M, Pan X, and Li X. 2013. "The environmental obesogen bisphenol A promotes adipogenesis by increasing the amount of 11 β-hydroxysteroid dehydrogenase type 1 in the adipose tissue of children." *International Journal of Obesity* (Lond) 37(7):999–1005. doi: 10.1038/ijo.2012.173.

17. Gump BB, Reihman J, Stewart P, Lonky E, Granger DA, and Matthews KA. 2009. "Blood lead (Pb) levels: further evidence for an environmental mechanism explaining the association between socio-economic status and psychophysiological dysregulation in children." *Health Psychology* 28(5):614–20. doi: 10.1037/a0015611.

18. Afaghi A, O'Connor H, and Chow CM. 2008. "Acute effects of the very low carbohydrate diet on sleep indices." *Nutritional Neuroscience* 11(4):146–54. doi: 10.1179/147683008X301540.

19. Jayson, S. 2012. "Stress levels increased since 1983, new analysis shows." *USA Today*, June 13. http://usatoday30.usatoday.com/news/health/story/2012–06–13/stress-increase-over-time/55587296/1.

20. Kubzansky LD, Bordelois P, Jun HJ, Roberts AL, Cerda M, Bluestone N, and Koenen KC. 2014. "The weight of traumatic stress: a prospective study of posttraumatic stress disorder symptoms and weight status in women." *JAMA Psychiatry* 71(1):44–51. doi: 10.1001/jamapsychiatry.2013.2798.

21. Tryon MS, DeCant R, and Laugero KD. 2013. "Having your cake and eating it too: a habit of comfort food may link chronic social stress exposure and acute stress-induced cortisol hyporesponsiveness." *Physiology and Behavior* 114–15:32–37. doi: 10.1016/j.physbeh.2013.02.018.

22. Kim Y, Yang HY, Kim AJ, and Lim Y. 2013. "Academic stress levels were positively associated with sweet food consumption among Korean high-school students." *Nutrition* 29(1):213–18. doi: 10.1016/j.nut.2012.08.005.

23. Yau YH, and Potenza MN. 2013. "Stress and eating behaviors." *Minerva Endocrinologica* 38(3):255–67.

CHAPTER 2

1. Vincent JM, Morrison ID, Armstrong P, and Reznek RH. 1994. "The size of normal adrenal glands on computed tomography." *Clinical Radiology* 49(7):453–55.

2. Morris, H. 2013. "Why stay in Chernobyl? Because it's home." *TED Talk*. Video. www.ted.com/talks/holly_morris_why_stay_in_chernobyl_because_it_s_home.html.

3. Hernandez-Morante JJ, Gomez-Santos C, Milagro F, Campión J, Martínez JA, Zamora S, and Garaulet M. 2009. "Expression of cortisol

metabolism-related genes shows circadian rhythmic patterns in human adipose tissue." *International Journal of Obesity* (Lond) 33(4):473–80. doi: 10.1038/ijo.2009.4.

4. Ibid.

5. Stimson RH, Mohd-Shukri NA, Bolton JL, Andrew R, Reynolds RM, and Walker BR. 2014. "The postprandial rise in plasma cortisol in men is mediated by macronutrient-specific stimulation of adrenal and extra-adrenal cortisol production." *Journal of Clinical Endocrinology and Metabolism* 99(1):160–68. doi: 10.1210/jc.2013–2307.

6. Tomlinson JW, Moore JS, Clark PM, Holder G, Shakespeare L, and Stewart PM. 2004. "Weight loss increases 11beta-hydroxysteroid dehydrogenase type 1 expression in human adipose tissue." *Journal of Clinical Endocrinology and Metabolism* 89(6):2711–16.

CHAPTER 3

1. Afaghi A, O'Connor H, and Chow CM. 2008. "Acute effects of the very low carbohydrate diet on sleep indices." *Nutritional Neuroscience* 11(4):146–54.

2. Flowers MT, and Ntambi JM. 2009. "Stearoyl-CoA desaturase and its relation to high-carbohydrate diets and obesity." *Biochimica et Biophysica Acta* 1791(2):85–91. doi: 10.1016/j.bbalip.2008.12.011.

3. Fischer K, Colombani PC, Langhans W, and Wenk C. 2002. "Carbohydrate to protein ratio in food and cognitive performance in the morning." *Physiology and Behavior* 75(3):411–23.

4. Dinneen S, Alzaid A, Miles J, and Rizza R. 1995. "Effects of the normal nocturnal rise in cortisol on carbohydrate and fat metabolism in IDDM." *American Journal of Physiology* 268(4 Pt 1):E595–603.

5. Kaczmarczyk MM, Miller MK, and Freund GG. 2012. "The health benefits of dietary fiber: beyond the usual suspects of type 2 diabetes mellitus, cardiovascular disease and colon cancer." *Metabolism* 61(8):1058–66. doi: 10.1016/j.metabol.0912.01.017.

6. Ibid.

7. Robertson MD, Bickerton AS, Dennis AL, Vidal H, and Frayn KN. 2005. "Insulin-sensitizing effects of dietary resistant starch and effects on skeletal muscle and adipose tissue metabolism." *American Journal of Clinical Nutrition* 82(3):559–67.

8. Kaprol M, Wawszczyk J, Smolik S, and Weglarz L. 2010. "Transcriptional regulation of interleukin 6 and its receptor in colon cancer cells by phytic acid." *Acta Poloniae Pharmaceutica* 67(6):701–705.

9. Bisschop PH, Sauerwein HP, Endert E, and Romijn JA. 2001. "Isocaloric carbohydrate deprivation induces protein catabolism despite a low T3-syndrome in healthy men." *Clinical Endocrinology* (Oxf) 54(1):75–80.

10. Bray GA, Smith SR, de Jonge L, Xie H, Rood J, Martin CK, Most M, Brock C, Mancuso S, and Redman LM. 2012. "Effect of dietary protein content on weight gain, energy expenditure, and body composition during overeating: a randomized controlled trial." *JAMA* 307(1):47–55. doi: 10.1001/jama.2011.1918.

11. Ibid.

12. Doerge DR, and Sheehan DM. 2002. "Goitrogenic and estrogenic activity of soy isoflavones." *Environmental Health Perspectives* 110 (Suppl 3):349–53.

CHAPTER 4

1. Gibson EL, Checkley S, Papadopoulos A, Poon L, Daley S, and Wardle J. 1999. "Increased salivary cortisol reliably induced by a protein-rich midday meal." *Psychosomatic Medicine* 61(2):214–24.

2. Anderson KE, Rosner W, Khan MS, New MI, Pang SY, Wissel PS, and Kappas A. 1987. "Diet-hormone interactions: protein/carbohydrate ratio alters reciprocally the plasma levels of testosterone and cortisol and their respective binding globulins in man." *Life Sciences* 40(18):1761–68.

3. Van Cauter E, Shapiro ET, Tillil H, and Polonsky KS. 1992. "Circadian modulation of glucose and insulin responses to meals: relationship to cortisol rhythm." *American Journal of Physiology* 262(4 Pt 1):E467–75.

CHAPTER 5

1. Grineva EN, Karonova T, Micheeva E, Belyaeva O, and Nikitina IL. 2013. "Vitamin D deficiency is a risk factor for obesity and diabetes type 2 in women at late reproductive age." *Aging* (Albany NY) 5(7):575–81.

2. Pinto JE. 1979. "The blocking effect of magnesium on the secretion of adrenal catecholamines induced by the omission of sodium from the extracellular medium." *Hormone and Metabolic Research* 11(6):404–407.

3. US Department of Agriculture. 2009. "CNMap Connecticut." Last modified April 22. www.ars.usda.gov/services/docs.htm?docid=11046.

4. Rayssiguier Y, Libako P, Nowacki W, and Rock E. 2010. "Magnesium deficiency and metabolic syndrome: stress and inflammation may reflect calcium activation." *Magnesium Research* 23(2):73–80. doi: 10.1684/mrh.2010.0208.

5. Sera N, Morita K, Nagasoe M, Tokieda H, Kitaura T, and Tokiwa H. 2005. "Binding effect of polychlorinated compounds and environmental carcinogens on rice bran fiber." *Journal of Nutritional Biochemistry* 16(1):50–58.

6. Thorn L, Hucklebridge F, Esgate A, Evans P, and Clow A. 2004. "The effect of dawn simulation on the cortisol response to awakening in healthy participants." *Psychoneuroendocrinology* 29(7):925–30.

7. Alvarez V, Maeder-Ingvar M, and Rosetti AO. 2011. "Watching television: a previously unrecognized powerful trigger of λ waves." *Journal of Clinical Neurophysiology* 28(4):400–403. doi: 10.1097/WNP.0b013e3182273250.

8. Ueno T, and Ohnaka T. 2006. "Influence of long-term exposure to an air-conditioned environment on the diurnal cortisol rhythm." *Journal of Physiological Anthropology* 25(6):357–62.

9. Harmer CJ, Charles M, McTavish S, Favaron E, and Cowen PJ. 2012. "Negative ion treatment increases positive emotional processing in seasonal affective disorder." *Psychological Medicine* 42(8):1605–12. doi: 10.1017/S0033291711002820.

10. Ryushi T, Kita I, Sakurai T, Yasumatsu M, Isokawa M, Aihara Y, and Hama K. 1998. "The effect of exposure to negative air ions on the recovery of physiological responses after moderate endurance exercise." *International Journal of Biometeorology* 41(3):132–36.

11. Goel N, and Etwaroo GR. 2006. "Bright light, negative air ions and auditory stimuli produce rapid mood changes in a student population: a placebo-controlled study." *Psychological Medicine* 36(9):1253–63.

CHAPTER 6

1. Harte JL, and Elfert GH. 1985. "The effects of running, environment, and attentional focus on athletes' catecholamine and cortisol levels and mood." *Psychophysiology* 32(1):49–54.

2. Olds TS, Maher CA, and Matricciani L. 2011. "Sleep duration or bedtime? Exploring the relationship between sleep habits and weight status and activity patterns." *Sleep* 34(10):1299–307. doi: 10.5665/SLEEP.1266.

3. Kripke DF, Langer RD, and Kline LE. 2012. "Hypnotics' association with mortality or cancer: a matched cohort study." *BMJ Open* 2(1):e000850. doi: 10.1136/bmjopen-2012-000850.

4. Storrs C. 2014. "13 Drugs That Can Make You Gain Weight." *Health*. Accessed February 11. www.health.com/health/gallery/thumbnails/0,,20545602,00.html.

5. Pawlow LA, and Jones GE. 2005. "The impact of abbreviated progressive muscle relaxation on salivary cortisol and salivary immunoglobulin A (sIgA)." *Applied Psychophysiology and Biofeedback* 30(4):375–87.

6. Kennedy DO, Little W, Haskell CF, and Scholey AB. 2006. "Anxiolytic effects of a combination of Melissa officinalis and Valeriana officinalis during laboratory induced stress." *Phytotherapy Research* 20(2):96–102.

7. Winston D, and Maimes S. 2007. *Adaptogens: Herbs for Strength, Stamina, and Stress Relief* (Vermont: Healing Arts Press).

8. Billioti de Gage S, Bégaud B, Bazin F, Verdoux H, Dartigues JF, Pérès K, Kurth T, and Pariente A. 2012. "Benzodiazepine use and risk of dementia: prospective population based study." *BMJ* 345:e6231. doi: 10.1136/bmj.e6231.

9. Wolfman C, Viola H, Paladini A, Dajas F, and Medina JH. 1994. "Possible anxiolytic effects of chrysin, a central benzodiazepine receptor ligand isolated from Passiflora coerulea." *Pharmacology Biochemistry and Behavior* 47(1):1–4.

10. Ngan A, and Conduid R. 2011. "A double-blind, placebo-controlled investigation of the effects of Passiflora incarnate (passionflower) herbal tea on subjective sleep quality." *Phytotherapy Research* 25(8):1153–59. doi: 10.1002/ptr.3400. Epub 2011 Feb 3.

CHAPTER 7

1. Kumari M, Shipley M, Stafford M, and Kivimaki M. 2011. "Association of diurnal patterns in salivary cortisol with all-cause and cardiovascular mortality: findings from the Whitehall II study." *Journal of Clinical Endocrinology and Metabolism* 96(5):1478–85. doi: 10.1210/jc.2010–2137.

2. Katagiri F, Inoue S, Sato Y, Itoh H, and Takeyama M. 2004. "Comparison of the effects of Sho-hange-ka-bukuryo-to and Nichin-to on human plasma adrenocorticotropic hormone and cortisol levels with continual stress exposure." *Biological and Pharmaceutical Bulletin* 27(10):1679–82.

3. Jitomir J, and Willoughby DS. 2009. "Cassia cinnamon for the attenuation of glucose intolerance and insulin resistance resulting from sleep loss." *Journal of Medicinal Food* 12(3):467–72. doi: 10.1089/jmf.2008.0128.

4. Anisimov VN, Vinogradova IA, Panchenko AV, Popovich IG, and Zabezhinski MA. 2012. "Light-at-night-induced circadian disruption, cancer and aging." *Current Aging Science* 5(3):170–77.

5. Panossian A, Wikman G, and Sarris J. 2010. "Rosenroot (Rhodiola rosea): traditional use, chemical composition, pharmacology and clinical efficacy." *Phytomedicine* 17(7):481–93. doi: 10.1016/j.phymed.2010.02.002.

6. Olsson EM, von Schéele B, and Panossian AG. 2009. "A randomised, double-blind, placebo-controlled, parallel-group study of the standardised extract shr-5 of the roots of Rhodiola rosea in the treatment of subjects with stress-related fatigue." *Planta Medica* 75(2):105–12. doi: 10.1055/s-0028-1088346.

7. Chandrasekhar K, Kapoor J, and Anishetty S. 2012. "A prospective, randomized double-blind, placebo-controlled study of safety and efficacy of a high-concentration full-spectrum extract of ashwagandha root in reducing stress and anxiety in adults." *Indian Journal of Psychological Medicine* 34(3):255–62. doi: 10.4103/0253-7176.106022.

CHAPTER 8

1. Lorenz MW, Markus HS, Bots ML, Rosvall M, and Sitzer M. 2007. "Prediction of clinical cardiovascular events with carotid intima-media thickness: a systematic review and meta-analysis." *Circulation* 115(4):459–67.

2. Biondo PD, Robbins SJ, Walsh JD, McCargar LJ, Harber VJ, and Field CJ. 2008. "A randomized controlled crossover trial of the effect of ginseng consumption on the immune response to moderate exercise in healthy sedentary men." *Applied Physiology, Nutrition, and Metabolism* 33(5):966–75. doi: 10.1139/H08–080.

3. Monograph. 2005. "Glycyrrhiza glabra." *Alternative Medicine Review* 10(3):230–37.

4. Amsterdam JD, Li Y, Soeller I, Rockwell K, Mao JJ, and Shuts J. 2009. "A randomized, double-blind, placebo-controlled trial of oral Matricaria recutita (chamomile) extract therapy for generalized anxiety disorder." *Journal of Clinical Psychopharmacology* 29(4):378–82. doi: 10.1097/JCP.0b013a3181ac935c.

CHAPTER 9

1. Keller A, Litzelman K, Wisk LE, Maddox T, Cheng ER, Creswell PD, and Witt WP. 2012. "Does the perception that stress affects health matter? The association with health and mortality." *Health Psychology* 31(5):677–84. doi: 10.1037/a0026743.

2. Adams S. 2012. "Why Winning Powerball Won't Make You Happy." *Forbes*, November 28. www.forbes.com/sites/susanadams/2012/11/28/why-winning-powerball-wont-make-you-happy/.

3. Sahakian BJ, Burdess C, Luckhurst H, and Trayhurn P. 1982. "Hyperactivity and obesity: the interaction of social isolation and cafeteria feeding." *Physiology and Behavior* 28(1):117–24.

4. Johnson C. 1999. "The Roseto Effect." Accessed February 11, 2014. www.uic.edu/classes/osci/osci590/14_2%20The%20Roseto%20Effect.htm.

5. Luks A, and Payne P. 2001. *The Healing Power of Doing Good* (Nebraska: iUniverse.com).

6. Piliavin JA, and Siegl E. 2007. "Health benefits of volunteering in the Wisconsin longitudinal study." *Journal of Health and Social Behavior* 48(4):450–64.

JUST THE FAQS

1. Akmal M, Khan SA, and Khan AQ. 2009. "The effect of the ALCAT test diet therapy for food sensitivity in patients with obesity." *Middle East Journal of Family Medicine* 7(3).

2. Krieger JW, Sitren HS, Daniels MJ, and Langkamp-Henken B. 2006. "Effects of variation in protein and carbohydrate intake on body mass and composition during energy restriction: a meta-regression." *American Journal of Clinical Nutrition* 83(2):260–74.

3. Winham DM, and Hutchins AM. 2011. "Perceptions of flatulence from bean consumption among adults in 3 feeding studies." *Nutrition* 10:128. doi: 10.1186/1475-2891-10-128.

index